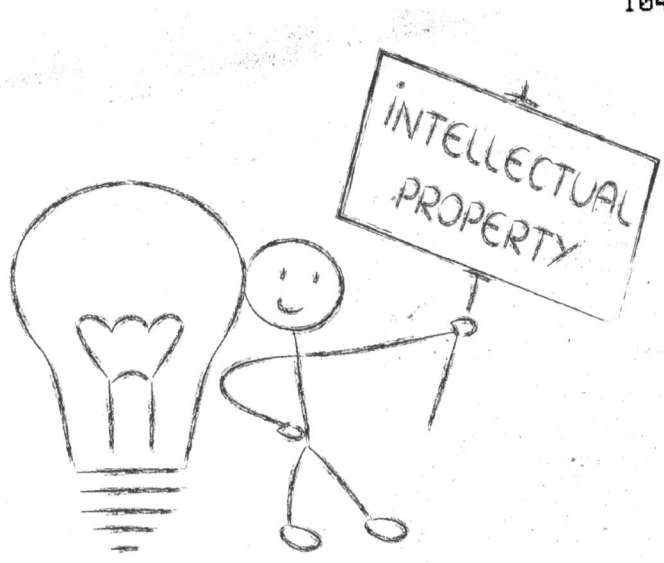

Table of Contents

Weight Watchers CookBook

There are several reasons for wanting to start a diet and want to lose weight. This may be after pregnancy or any excessive weight gain, and this may simply be meant to seduce or feel better in one's body. But this can also be for medical reasons. Excess weight can cause problems. Joint problems, heart or arterial problems.

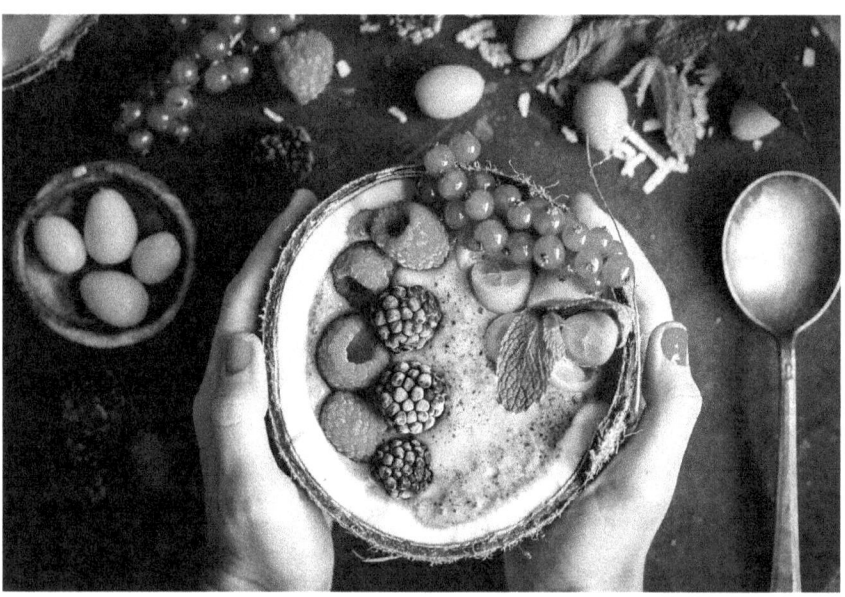

Before starting a diet, it is important to know where you are going and where you want to go.

Body Mass Index (BMI)

BMI is a theoretical and empirical index calculated from height and weight to evaluate whether one is overweight. The variables in this index are mainly morphological and should weigh the result.

Therefore, the purely statistical BMI is calculated as follows:

Bodyweight (kilograms) divided by height (meters squared)

$$BMI = x \, KG / (y \, M * y \, M)$$
x=bodyweight in KG
y=height in m

The result can be found in the following categories:

- *Less than 18: too lean*
- *Between 18 and 25: ideal weight*
- *Between 25 and 30: overweight*
- *More than 30: obesity*
- *Beyond 35: morbid obesity*

How fast do you lose weight?

The speed at which one loses weight depends on different parameters. Physical activity, food, social activities, gender, etc.

Nevertheless, it is generally observed that too rapid a loss leads to an equally rapid recovery. And on the other hand, it is quite normal to lose much more the first few weeks. You can imagine losing 1 kilo a week during the first month and 500 grams per week the following months.

Set goals

In order to follow your progress, it is important to establish a starting point, an end point and possibly intermediate steps (especially if the desired loss is more than 10 kilos). The best thing is to note regularly the ideal weight under the same conditions and this can be once a week: in the morning, after having been to the toilet, before breakfast, and in the same attire.

Different types of diets

There are several methods of weight loss based on diet. We have the ketogenic diet, paleo diet, vegan, etc. In this book, we are going to major on the Weight Watchers diet. With this diet, you can consume anything that you want.This popular weight reduction plan has been revised, and the fundamental policy of eating what you love still remains - although the diet program steers you towards healthier and nutritious foods with its point system.

Weight Watchers is not just a diet but a lifestyle-changing plan. It can help you master how to eat better and engage in more physical activities so that you can lose weight.

What you can eat and what you cannot.

There isn't any type food that is banned if you follow the weight watchers plan. Weight Watchers assign different types of foods to a SmartPoints value, which in turn replenishes its long-standing Points-Plus program. However, the concept is the same. The diet plan now factors fats, sugar, and protein to control you towards lean proteins, fruits, vegetables, and away from things that are high in sugars and saturated fats.

Weight watchers smartpoints for most tracked foods.

- Milk, skim (fat free), 1 cup (3SP)
- Strawberries (0SP)
- Egg, 1 (2 SP)
- Apple (0SP)
- Butter, 1 tbsp. (5SP)
- Watermelon (0SP)
- Egg white, 1 (0SP)
- Lettuce (0SP)
- Cooked Bacon 3 slices (5SP)
- Milk, reduced fat 2%, 1 cup (5SP)
- Red wine, 5 ounces (4SP)
- Water (0SP)
- Oatmeal, cooked, 1 cup (5SP)
- Almonds, 1/4 cup (4SP)

- Black coffee, black, without sugar, 1 cup (0SP)
- 3 ounces cooked and boneless chicken breast, 3 ounces (2SP)
- Grapes (0SP)
- Avocado, Hass, 1/4 (2SP)
- Carrots, baby (0SP)
- Orange (0SP)
- Milk, low fat 1%, 1 cup (4SP)
- Cheddar or colby cheese, 1 ounce (4SP)
- White sugar, 1 teaspoon (1SP)
- Almond milk,

- Banana (0 SP)
- Salad, mixed greens (0SP)
- Blueberries (0S)
- Tomatoes (0SP)
- Olive oil, 1 tablespoon (4SP)
- Half cream, tablespoons (2SP)
- Bread, 1 slice (2SP)
- Deli turkey, 2 ounces (1SP)
- Cucumber (0SP)
- Broccoli (0SP)
- White rice, 1 cup (6SP)
- Pineapple (0S)
- Green beans (0SP)
- White wine, 5 ounces (4SP)

- Egg, fried, 1 (3SP)
- Tortilla chips, 1 ounce (4SP)
- Fruit, fresh, unsweetened (0SP)
- Raspberries (0SP)
- Cooked shrimp, 3 ounces (1 SP)
- Celery (0SP)
- Asparagus (0SP)
- Sweet Potatoes, 1/2 cup (3SP)
- American cheese, 1 ounce (4SP)
- Sweet red peppers (0SP)
- Salad dressing, low fat balsamic vinaigrette, 1 tbsp. (1SP)
- Hamburger bun, 1 or 2 ounces (5SP)
- Tuna fish, canned and

- plain, unsweetened, 1 cup (1SP)
- Cherries (0SP)
- Spinach (0SP)
- Potato, baked, plain, 1, 6 ounces (5SP)
- Peanut butter, 2 tbsps. (6SP)
- Honey, 1 tbsp. (4SP)
- English muffin, 2 ounces (4SP)
- Greek yogurt, plain, fat-free, 1 cup (3SP)
- fat-free salsa (0SP)
- cooked Pasta or wheat, 1 cup (5SP)
- Hummus, 2 tablespoons (2SP)
- Cherry tomatoes (0SP)
- Pear (0SP)
- Feta, crumbled, 1 ounce (3SP)

- Brown rice, cooked, 1 cup (6SP)
- Corn on the cob, 1 medium (4SP)
- Cantaloupe (0SP)
- Mayonnaise, 1 tablespoon (3SP)
- Carrots (0SP)
- meat, ham, honey, lean, 2 ounces (2SP)
- homemade Cookies, chocolate, oatmeal, 1 or 1/2 ounce (3SP)
- Peach (0SP)
- Pork chop, cooked, lean, 3 ounces (3SP)
- Mushrooms (0SP)
- Mashed potatoes, 1/2 cup (4SP)
- Tortilla, flour, 1 medium or 1 ounce (3SP)

- drained, 3 ounces (1SP)
- Ground beef, 90% lean, 3 ounces (4SP)
- Berries, mixed (0SP)
- Mango (0SP)
- Grapefruit (0SP)
- French fries, 20 or 5.5 ounces (13SP)
- Salad dressing, ranch, 2 tablespoons (5SP)
- Cottage cheese, fat-free, 1 cup (2SP)

- Canned black beans, 1/2 cup (3SP)
- Zucchini (0SP)
- Diet Coke, 8 ounces (0SP)
- Milk, whole, 1 cup (7SP)
- Guacamole, 2 tablespoons, (1SP)
- Italian Salad dressing, (not creamy), 2 tablespoons (3SP)

- Onions (0SP)
- Blackberries (0SP)
- Nectarine (0SP)
- Bagel, 1 small or 1/2 large, 2 ounces (5SP)
- Turkey bacon, cooked, 3 slices (3SP)
- Grape tomatoes (0SP)
- Mustard, 1 tablespoon (0SP)

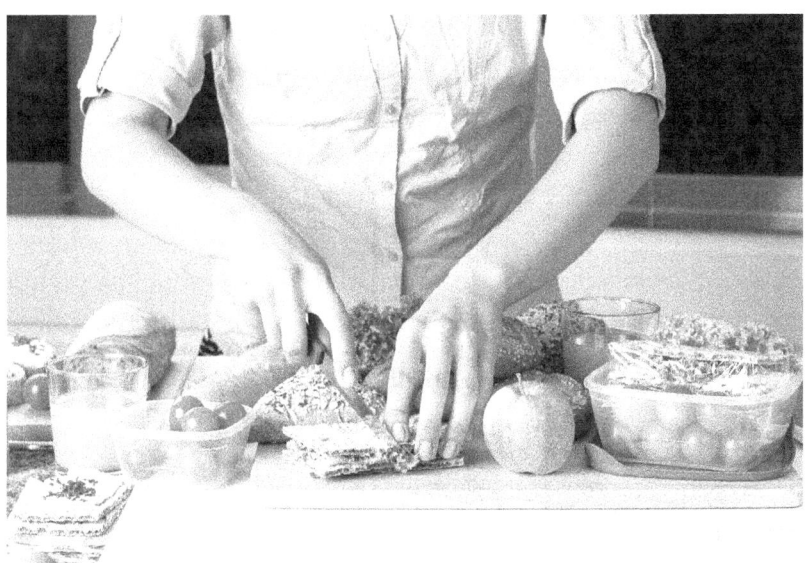

Apples

"An apple a day keeps the doctor away" You must have heard this simple phrase in your childhood thousand times! So eat an apple every day and its phytonutrients, antioxidants and dietary fiber will keep you slim and fit. You can eat an apple anytime.

Oats

Carbohydrates found in oats are very useful in terms of releasing hormone serotonin which burns fat faster than any other thing. Moreover, it provides relaxation. You can add them in your meals and enjoy it.

Yoghurt

Yoghurt is one of the most easily digestible in comparison to milk. Calcium and Vitamin-B are one of the most important part of its properties that are known for boosting immunity. It also helps for increases hunger. Yoghurt is a kind of medicine available at your home that you must use to prevent blood sugar and colon cancer.

Pomegranate

Pomegranates provide us a lot fiber. Moreover, pomegranates are rich source of antioxidants and folic acid. Pomegranates are fantastic alternative for sugar. Try it and satisfy your sugar cravings.

Lentils

Lentils are very good source of protein and fiber. In addition to it lentils also offer us marvelous resistant starch fiber (a kind of carbohydrate that improves our metabolic process and burns unnecessary fat).

Green tea

Do you drink tea containing caffeine? Well if your answer is yes than you need to switch to green tea immediately. Switching to green tea's 2-3 cups a day not only enhances your fat burning process via antioxidants present in it but also reduces your weight faster than your expectations.

Watermelon

Water is the most dominating property of watermelon. It has 92% water and Vitamin A and C also to fuel weight loss naturally. It is wonderful in taste and also good for satisfying your thirst in scorching hot summer days.

So these are some of the super foods that you can include in your diet and trigger weight loss to get back to your old shape. However, we strongly recommend you to consult your doctor before using this information for Weight Loss because he knows your body the best.

CALORIE TABLE

This table provides a calorie break down of all the foods mentioned in this book.

FOOD	WEIGHT(grams)/Unit	Calories
Apples	100	64
Apricot	30	19
Banana	100	120
Bean soup	300	289
Beet	35	17
Broccoli	60	22
Avocado	146	243
Strawberries	10	4
Brussel sprouts	100	59
Cabbage	30	8
Cauliflower	80	25
Cucumber	150	22
Egg plant	30	6
Fruit salad	150	230
Grape	150	118

Garlic	5	7
Hazelnut	3	19
Kale	50	13
Lemons	60	22
Lentils	120	152
lettuce	35	6
Mushroom	80	15
Mangos	260	182
Melon	100	30
Olive	5	11
Oranges	100	43
Peaches	100	90
Pears	20	18
Peas	20	18
Pine nuts	10	22
Pineapple	100	52
Pineapple syrup	150	184
radish	10	2
Raisin	100	28
Red plum	50	27

Spinach	80	18
Tangerine	100	50
Tomato	100	25
Turnips	100	35
Vegetable soup	300	215
watercress	25	6
Water melon	100	31
Almond	3	19
Bean casserole	300	456
Cooked brown rice	40	45
Cooked white rice	40	44
Corn	20	25
Corn flour	20	73
Corn starch	20	69
Oat flakes	15	49
Wheat	20	72
Wheat flour	20	75
Muffins	90	12
Pies: Apple Blue berry	295	43

Mayonnaise	60	4
Coffee/tea	1 cup	26
Chicken	100	252
Beef	100	313
Pork	100	252
Ham	100	242
Salmon	100	194
Crab	100	82
Tuna	100	130

BREAKFAST RECIPES

Slow Cooker Cocktail Smokies

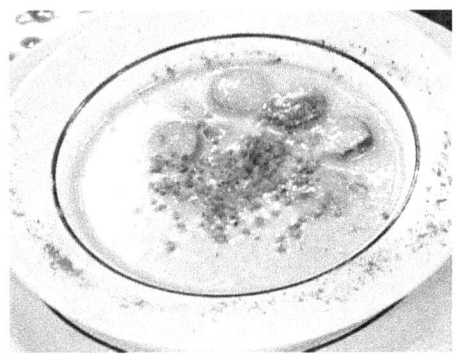

Ready in 2 h. 10 mins.

8 servings.

Ingredients

- 2 (16 ounce) packages cocktail beef sausages
- 1 (12 ounce) bottle barbeque sauce
- 1 (8 ounce) jar of jelly grape

Preparation

1. Combine the grape jelly with barbeque sauce in a slow cooker

2. Stir in the beef sausage cocktail

3. Cook on high heat until cooked for about two hours

4. Allow to cool for about 5 minutes before serving

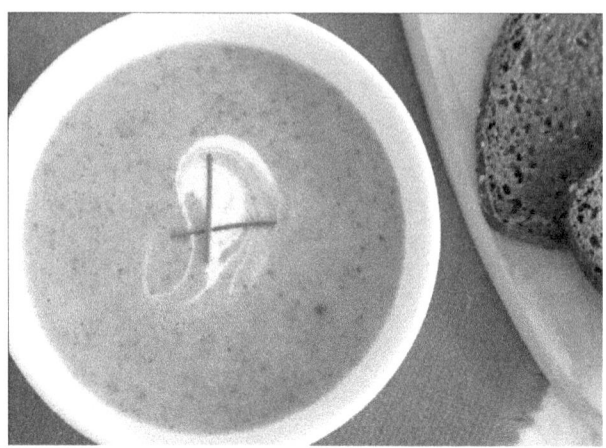

Prep time 6mins.
Cooking time 22min.
5 servings.

Ingredients
- 400 g broccoli, washed and chopped
- 200 gr of zucchini cut into dice
- 1 leek
- 50g butter
- Salt pepper
- Cheese

Preparation:
1. In a pan put the butter to melt, add the leek cut and melt. Then add the chopped vegetables, mixing well.
2. Wet vegetables until almost cover and cook for twenty minutes. Vegetables should be melting.
3. Mix everything with cheese to make a soup, salt and pepper and enjoy!

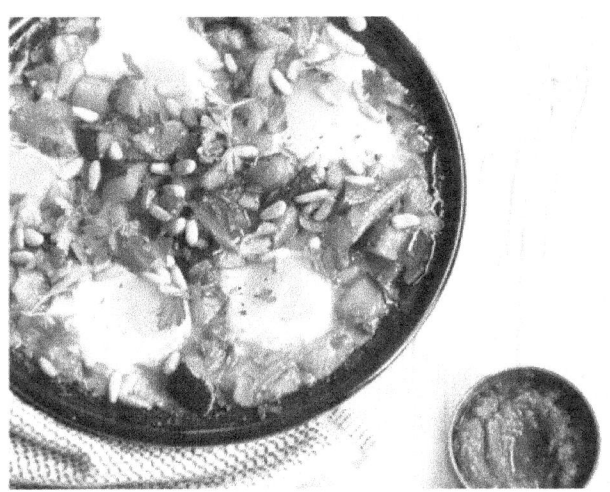

Prep time 5mins.

Cooking time 30min.

4 servings.

Ingredients

- 1 kg of lamb cut into the shoulder
- 1 chopped onion
- 1 large tomato, peeled, seeded and chopped
- 2 cloves garlic, minced
- 1 c. freshly ground black pepper
- 1 c. Coffee ginger
- 1 c. Coffee turmeric
- 4 cl oil
- 1 bunch coriander and parsley
- Salt
- Water
- For the vegetables:
- Oil for frying

Preparation

1. In a pot over low heat, Place the pieces of meat and add onion, garlic, tomatoes, spices, salt and oil. Fry for about 10 minutes. Moisten up with water, cover the pot and bring to boil.

2. After boiling, add the bouquet of herbs and cook it all under cover and over low heat.

3. Wash the eggplant and detail in 1.5 cm thick slices.

4. Salt the eggplant slices and let drain for 10 minutes, rinse, squeeze between the palms and pat dry.

5. When the meat and chickpeas are cooked (fluxes) and the reduced sauce, remove the bouquet of coriander and parsley.

6. In a serving dish, prepare the meat, cover with sauce and garnish with fried eggplant.

7. Serve hot tagine.

Banana chips

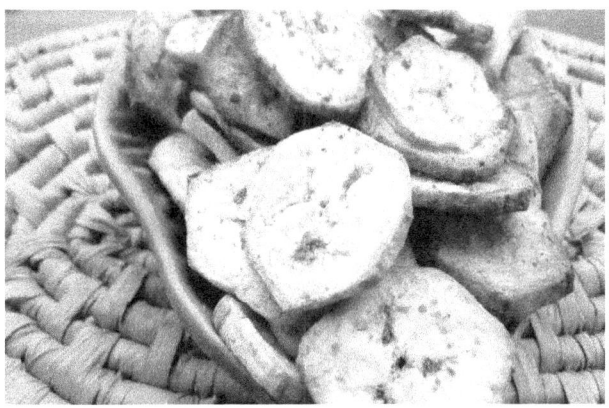

Ready after 20 minutes,

2 servings

Ingredients

- Black pepper
- Small amount Oil
- Salt
- 4 raw bananas

Preparation

1. Get the bananas peeled then make thin chips like slices by slicing them. Add a little oil to mix with the chips.

2. Setting the Airfryer at 180 degrees F, transfer the banana chips to the Airfryer.

3. Air fry for ten minutes then season with pepper and salt.

Cheese rice balls

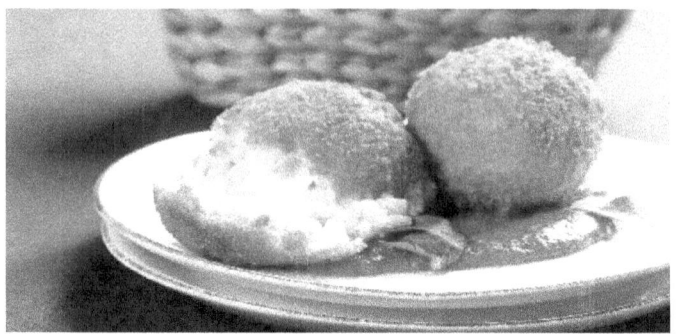

Ready after 40 minutes

6 servings

Ingredients

- 1 spoon Corn Flour Slurry

- 1 cup Paneer

- 2 spoons of Sweet Corn

- 1 spoon Corn Flour

- Bread Crumbs

- 1 finely chopped Green Chilly

- Garlic Powder (not a must)

- Small cubes of Mozzarella Cheese

- Oregano or Italian Seasoning

- 2 spoons of Carrot

- Salt

- 1 cup Boiled Rice

Preparation

1. Make dough using salt, corn flour, rice, paneer and seasoning in a bowl. Add chilly, cheese cubes, carrots, and sweet corn and make a good mixture.

2. Make balls of the stuffed dough and put the balls into corn slurry after which you roll the balls in bread crumbs and air fry them in the Airfryer preheated to 200 degrees F.

3. Best when served hot.

McCain Veggie fingers

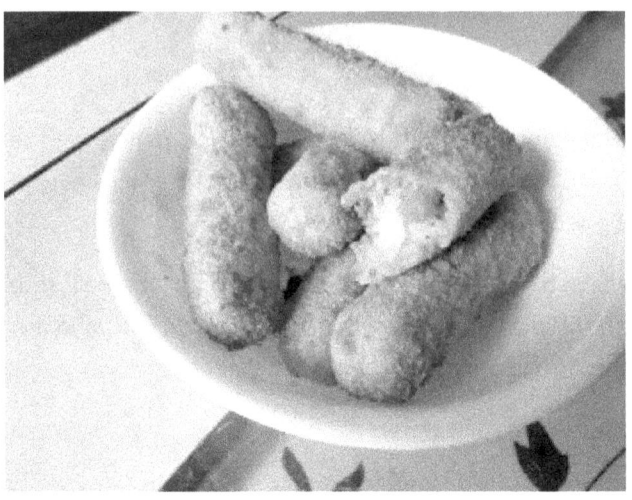

Ready after 20 minutes

6 servings

Ingredients

- Frozen veggie fingers (as many as desired)

Preparation

1. Get the veggie fingers out of the freezer.

2. Place them in the Airfryer and allow them to cook for twenty minutes until they are crispy.

Pasta parcel

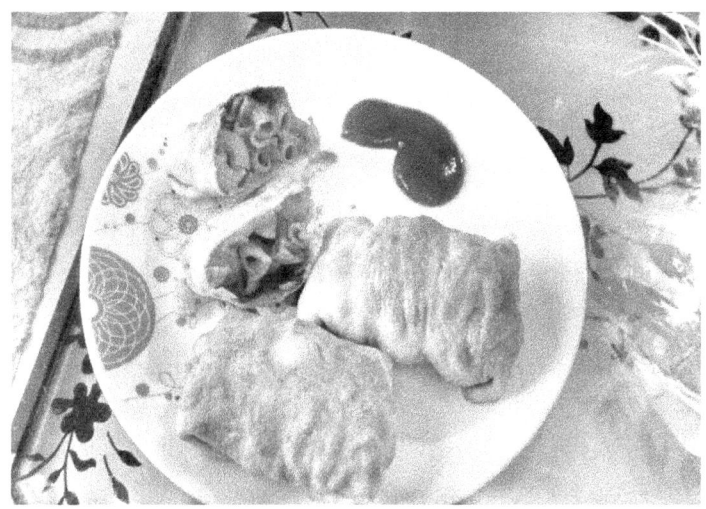

Ready after 20 minutes

6 servings

Ingredients

- 1 cup of flour
- Salt
- ¼ cup tomato paste
- 2 chopped onions
- 1 teaspoon garam masala
- 1 cup of water
- 2 tablespoons of oil
- 2 pieces of green chili

Preparation

1. Make a mixture of salt, water and 1 cup flour then keep aside after applying a little oil.

2. Boil the pasta with one tablespoon oil and salt then get rid of any excess.

3. Cook green chili, salt, garam masala, tomato paste and chopped onions and add pasta then cover and cook on low heat.

4. Using a rolling pin, make circles out of the dough balls. Get the edges sealed using water then get them cooked in the Airfryer for 15 minutes at 200 degrees F. Cook up to the point they are golden brown.

Cheese spinach balls

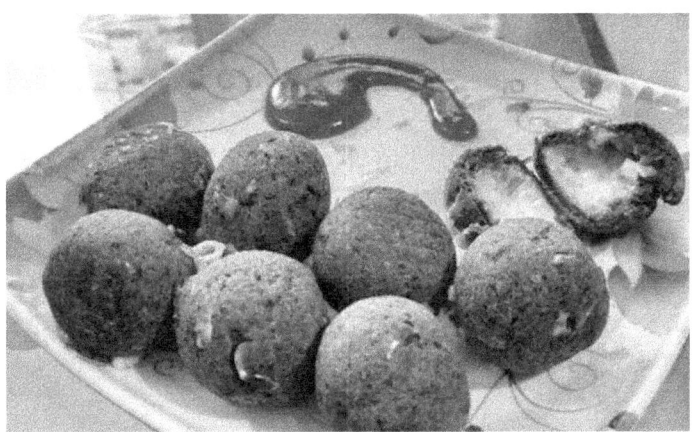

Ready after 30 minutes

6 servings

Ingredients

- Bread crumbs
- Red chili flakes
- 1 cup Corn flour
- 2 tablespoons of Oil
- Grated garlic
- 1 tablespoon of Salt
- 2 small chopped onions
- Mozzarella cheese (grated)

Preparation

1. Make a paste of bread crumbs, corn flour, and boiled spinach, some salt, grated mozzarella and garlic. Make the paste into balls.

2. Make small balls out of a mixture of chili flakes, onions and cheese fillings.

Use your oil to brush the balls then air fry them for fifteen minutes with the Airfryer at 200 F

Quiche without crust

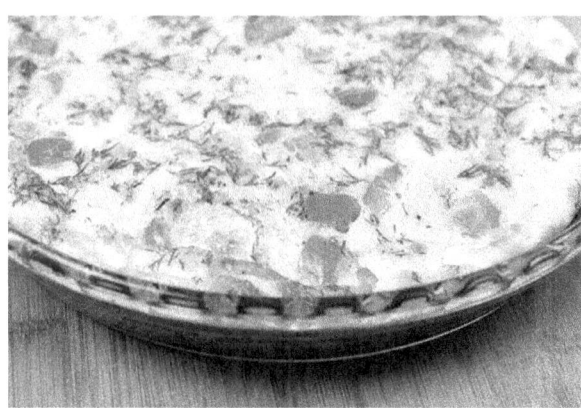

Prep time 5mins.

Cooking time 20min.

3 portions.

Ingredients

- 8 eggs
- 1 bowl of fresh cream
- 1 bowl of grated cheese
- Salt and pepper
- 1 clove of garlic, minced
- Filling: 100 gr fried mushrooms, 100 or 100 gr shrimp cooked ground meat and 100 grams of peppers, or cooked chicken breast and 100 gr feta ....

Preparation

1. Beat eggs with cream, chopped clove of garlic, salt and pepper in a bowl.

2. Place the toppings of your choice into muffin molds and pour over eggs preparedness.

3. Bake at 180 degrees for 15 minutes.

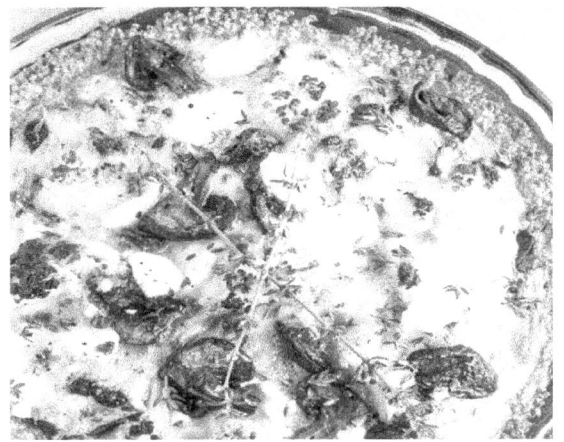

Prep time 5mins.

Cooking time 20min.

8 portions.

Ingredients

- A cauliflower half-head
- 200 grams of paris mushrooms
- 6 eggs
- 5 cl fresh cream
- A clove of minced garlic
- 2 tablespoons of chopped chives coffee
- 50g butter
- 100g grated cheese
- Salt and pepper

Preparation

1. Cook the cauliflower steamed, cool and mash with a fork.

2. Fry the sliced mushrooms in butter. Mix with remaining ingredients and place in muffin tins.

Corn on the cob

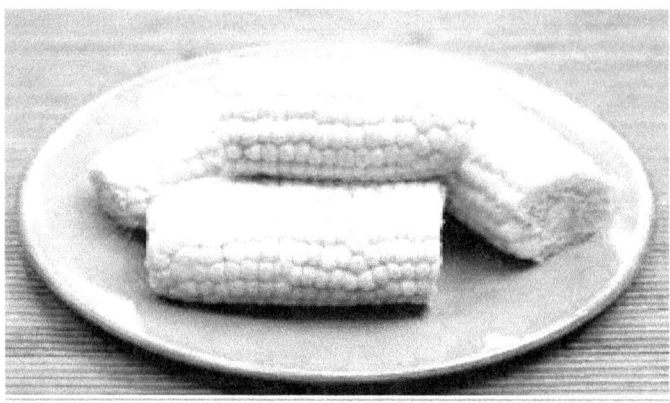

Preparation time: 5 minutes| cooking time: 12 minutes | serve for 5

Ingredients

- 8 ears of corn

- 2 cups of water

- A pinch of salt

Preparation

1. Remove the corn from its husk and cut the bottom. Wash them thoroughly.

2. Add water to the pressure cooker and arrange the corn vertically with most of the corn covered by water leaving only a small end up. If the ear is too elongated lay it horizontally. Do not overcrowd the corns to let them cook well.

3. Lock the lid firmly on the pressure cooker. For electric cookers cook for 2 minutes at high pressure while for stove cookers, let the corn cook under high hit for the first few minutes then lower the heat towards the end.

4. After the time stated above uncover the pressure cooker with the normal release.

5. Serve with lots of salt and butter.

LUNCH RECIPES

Kale masala

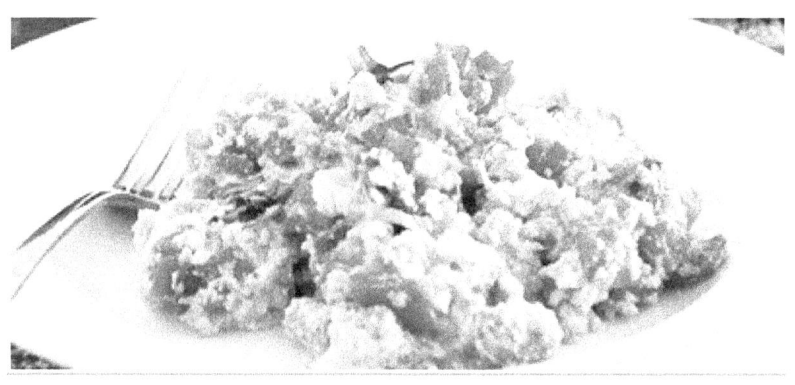

Ready in 30mins.

4 servings.

Ingredients

- 1 cup curly kale
- 30 ml of freshly chopped red onion
- Zest of one lemon
- 2-3 tablespoons lemon juice
- ¼ cup of chia seed
- Cumin seeds
- Coriander seeds
- Mustard seeds
- Black peppercorns
- Cayenne pepper

Preparation

1. Start by cleaning the kale leaves and remove stems and cut them into thin strips.
2. Take the zest of a lemon before squeezing and mix 2-3 tablespoons of lemon juice with fresh ground spices and lemon zest.
3. Pour this mixture over the kale, add the red onion and massage to soften the cabbage.
4. Divide the mixture obtained on a dehydrator tray and dry at 41 ° C for 12 to 24 hours. The mixture should be completely dry.
5. Upon exiting the dehydrator, you are left only to the dry the preparation in your food processor with chia seeds and mix to obtain a green powder.
6. Keep your green powder in a mason jar away from moisture, heat, and sprinkle!
7. Feel free to make your own mixes by choosing your spices and your favorite green leaves!

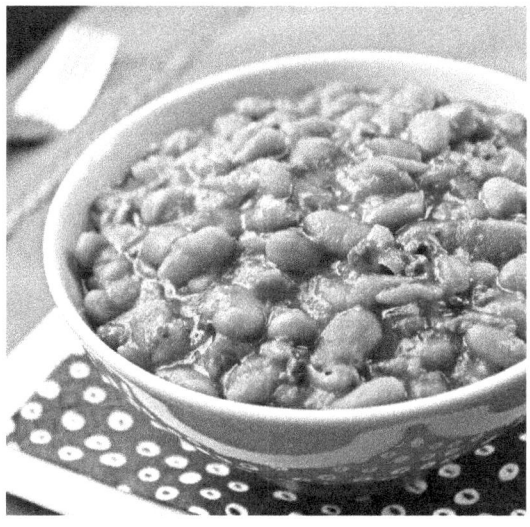

Ready in 5h. 15mins.

6 servings.

Ingredients:

- 2 cups of beans

- ½ pound (225 grams) of salt pork, diced

- 1 medium onion, whole

- ¼ cup (125 mL) brown sugar

- ¼ cup (125 mL) molasses

- 1 teaspoon (5 mL) dry mustard

- ¼ cup (125 mL) ketchup

- Pepper

Preparation:

1. Soak the beans overnight in a bowl of water with ½ teaspoon baking soda tea

2. The next day, rinse them, put them in a saucepan and boil in water for 30 minutes

3. Discard the water. Pour into slow cooker with bacon, onion in the center, pour sauce (brown sugar, molasses, mustard, ketchup) on the beans

4. Cover with hot water on high 1 hour and at low for 5 hours.

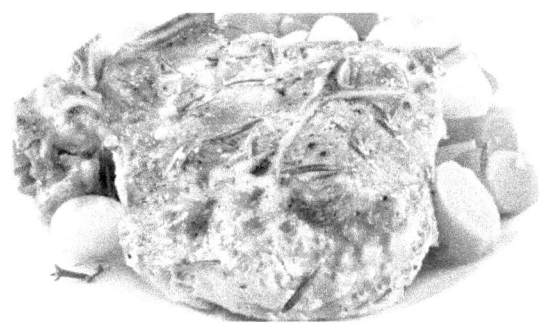

Ready in 8h. 15 mins.

6 servings.

Ingredients:

- Roast 1 pallet of about 2 lbs. calf
- 5-6 cloves garlic
- Dijon mustard
- Bovril chicken
- 1 consumed box
- 1 box of cream of mushroom

Preparation:

1. Prick the roast with garlic cloves, peeled and cut into pieces.
2. Mix a bit of Dijon mustard with Bovril and baste roast both sides.
3. Sear in a hot pan with a little butter and oil, the 2 sides.
4. Put the piece of meat in slow cooker.
5. In a bowl, mix the cream and consumed champignons.
6. Cook on low 8 hours.

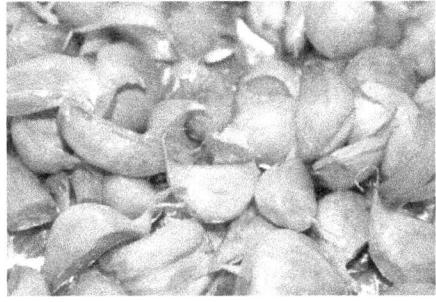

Ultimate fried English meal

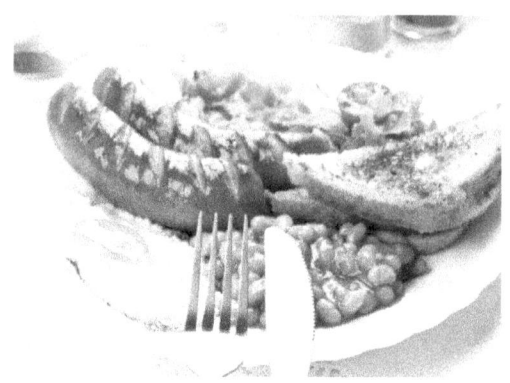

Ready after 25 minutes

4 servings

Ingredients

- 1 can of baked beans
- 8 rashers of unsmoked back bacon
- 8 slices toast
- 4 eggs
- 8 medium sausages

Preparation

1. Place the bacon and sausages in the Airfryer at 160 degrees F and allow them to cook for ten minutes.

2. Place the baked beans in one ramekins place and the egg in another.

3. On 200 degrees F, cook until it is all cooked through. You can serve.

Mishmash

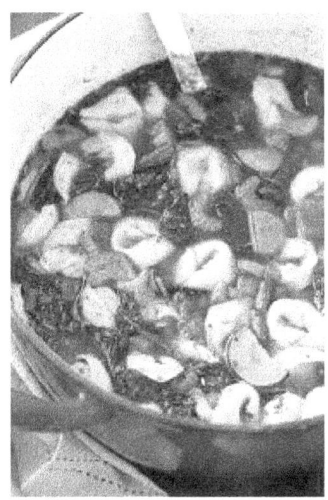

Ready in 5 minutes.

1 serving

Ingredients

- 1 medium tomato (120g)
- 1/2 avocado (70 g)
- 4 strawberries (50 g)
- 1 small handful of arugula
- White or black pepper to taste

Preparation:

1. Wash and cut into wedges and slices the diced tomato, avocado and strawberries.

2. Add chopped or whole rocket if the leaves are young and tender, then mix.

3. Remove nicely on a plate and fill with a few grinds of pepper.

4. Serve immediately or refrigerate for a very fresh tasting.

Vegetable tortellini soup

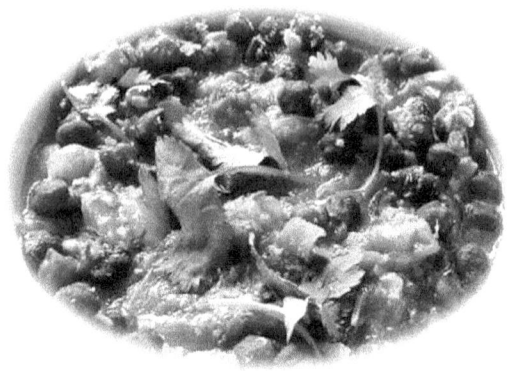

Ready after 25 minutes

4 servings

Ingredients

- 3 cups vegetable stock

- ½ cup of carrot

- ¼ cup finely chopped onions

- Pepper & salt, to taste

- 1/8 cup finely chopped leek

- ½ cup dried tortellini

- Parmesan cheese

- ½ cup courgettes

Preparation

1. Cut the courgettes into two then get the carrots peeled into small cubes.

2. Place the ingredients into the Airfryer since it serves in this case as your soup maker.

3. Cook while the lid is covered.

4. After about fifteen minutes of cooking under low heat, use parmesan cheese for garnishing.

Roast garlic and honey pallet

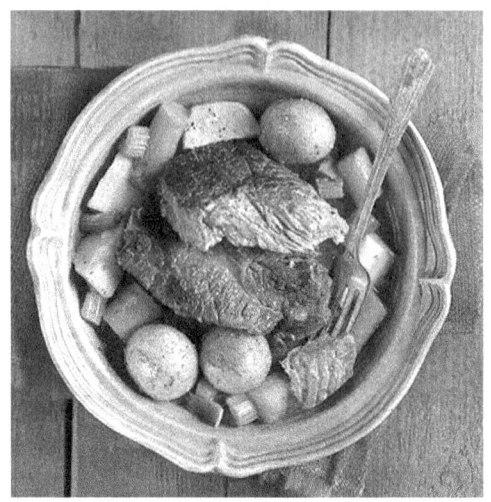

Ready in 8 h. 10mins.

6 servings.

Ingredients:

- 1 roast palette
- 1/2 bottle of 341 ml of VH Honey Garlic Cooking Sauce
- 1 box of 10 ounces beef broth
- Pepper

Preparation:

1. Put the roast in the slow cooker, add the consommé, the VH sauce and pepper well.
2. Cook on low for 8 hours.
3. For baking, cover and cook at 350 ° between 2 and 3 hours.

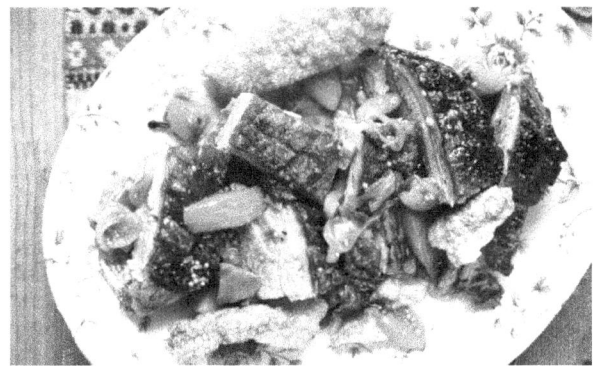

Ready in 8h. 30mins.

6 servings.

Ingredients:

- 1 lb. pork stew cube
- 1 c. Tablespoons oil
- 1 onion, quartered
- 1 small turnip cubes
- 1-2 cloves finely chopped garlic?
- 3 sliced carrots
- 3 stalks celery cut into chunks
- 1 cup beans green fees (my addition)
- 2 large potatoes cut into cubes (my addition)
- ¾ cup frozen peas (omitted)
- ½ cup of beer
- 1 ½ cups chicken broth
- 1 tbsp. brown sugar
- 2 tbsp. tablespoon Worcestershire sauce (custard)
- 2 tbsp. teaspoon thyme
- Salt and pepper

Preparation:

1. Coat the pork cubes and shake off excess.

2. Heat the oil in a heavy pot on medium-high heat.

3. Fry the pork and onion for 3-4 minutes?.

4. Add vegetables and cook 4-5 minutes.

5. Add the remaining ingredients.

6. Cover and simmer over low heat for 45 minutes. Season to taste.

7. Coat the pork cubes and shake off excess.

8. Heat oil in a pan over a medium-high heat. Brown the pork and onion for 3-4 minutes.

9. Place vegetables and liquid in the dish stoneware crock pot, add pork cubes and cook on low 8 hours.

Chili con carne

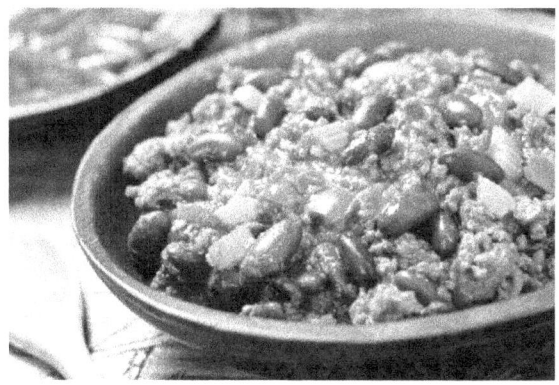

Prep time 5mins.

Cooking time 1h 10min.

6 servings.

Ingredients

- 750 grams of minced meat with fat

- 1 medium onion

- 3 green peppers

- 3 tablespoons tomato paste

- 1 tomato, diced

- 1 tablespoon Mexican seasoning

- 2 garlic clove

- 5 cl olive oil

- Salt and pepper

Preparation

- ✓ Cut the onion and diced peppers, crush the garlic and fry in a pan with half of the olive oil

- ✓ Fry the minced meat, salt and pepper in a pan.

- ✓ Add the chopped tomatoes and diced tomato paste to the pot with the Mexican seasoning, the rest of the olive oil and cooked ground meat.

- ✓ Cook everything over very low heat for one hour.

Queso fundido meat

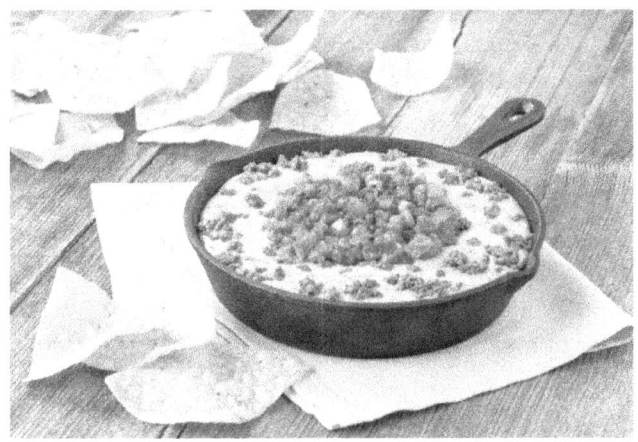

Prep time 5mins.

Cooking time 30min.

6 servings.

Ingredients

- 200 grams of minced meat
- A small onion knife
- 1 bowl of green peppers, yellow red e diced
- 200 grams of grated mozzarella
- 200 grams of grated Cheddar or Edam
- A pinch of pepper
- 1 tomato diced
- 3 tablespoons chopped cilantro
- 2 tbsp. olive oil
- 1 clove garlic, chopped

Preparation

- ✓ Preheat oven to 200 °. Fry salted minced meat and pepper in a pan with a tablespoons olive oil. Remove from heat and reserve the meat.

- ✓ In the same skillet, pour a tablespoon of olive oil, a clove of minced garlic, onion and peppers, cook until the onion becomes translucent. It should not be any liquid in the pan.

- ✓ In a baking dish (a cast iron skillet, or fried for paella), place a layer of meat, vegetables and cheese mixture. Place a last layer of cheese and sprinkle with pepper.

- ✓ Bake 10 minutes. We need the cheese melts completely but it does not take it begins to harden. At the exit of the oven decorate with crushed tomatoes and chopped coriander.

- ✓ Serve

Polenta and beans

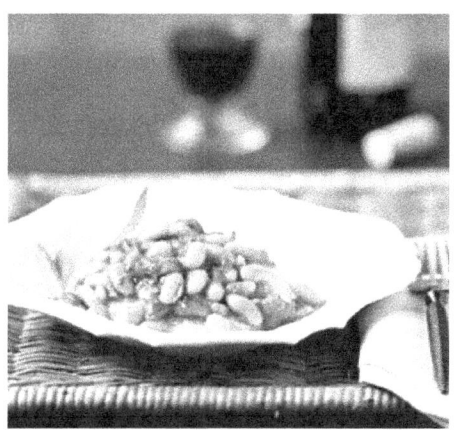

Prep time: 15 min

Cooking time: 1 h

6 servings

Ingredients

- 1 tablespoon leaf parsley
- 1 teaspoon chopped fresh sage
- 2 garlic cloves, minced
- 1 can diced tomatoes
- 1 (19-ounce) can cannellini beans, rinsed and drained
- 4 cups of water
- 1/2 teaspoon salt
- 2 tablespoons extra virgin olive oil
- 1 cup coarse yellow dry polenta
- 1/4 teaspoon freshly ground black pepper

Preparation

1. Heat olive oil in a pressure cooker under low heat. Add garlic and parsley and cook for 60 seconds. Add tomatoes and sage and cook until all liquid evaporates. That could mean 10 minutes.

2. Add to a pan 1/8 teaspoon salt, black pepper, and beans. Adjust to high pressure and cover then while stirring cook for six minutes.

3. Boil ½ teaspoon salt and 4 cups of water and add, in a thin stream and as you stir, polenta. Cook as you stir constantly for about 3 minutes. Cook for ten minutes while keeping it covered. Get off the cover and cook for two minutes. Cover again and cook for 6 minutes then get it uncovered again and cook for two minutes as you constantly stir. Pour water over the cooker at the sink for quick pressure release. You can now serve you polenta preferably with bean mixture.

Cauliflower cream

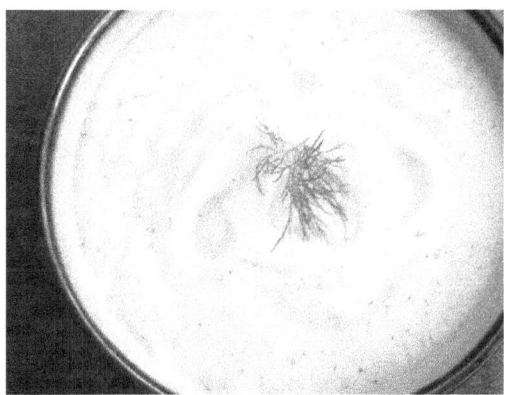

Prep time 8mins.

Cooking time 25min.

3 servings.

Ingredients

- 1 medium cauliflower

- 1 half onion

- Half a box of Philadelphia or Jebly herb

- 50g butter

- Salt and pepper

- 1 liter chicken stock

Preparation

1. Put the butter melt in a pan, add half onion and cauliflower cut pieces. Add salt and pepper, cover with broth.

2. Cook 20 minutes from the rotation of the valve.

3. Mix everything with Philadelphia cheese with herbs.

Fried chicken with coconut flour

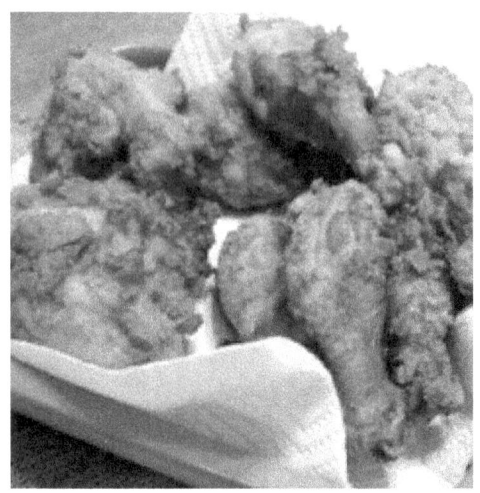

Prep time 5mins.

Cooking time 20min.

6 servings.

Ingredients

- 2 kg of chicken thighs (up and pestle)

- Salt pepper

- Garlic powder or two garlic cloves mashed

- 1 tablespoon paprika

- 100 grams of coconut flour

- Oil for frying

Preparation

1. Marinade: In a large bowl, combine the chicken, salt, pepper, garlic and paprika. Mix well with your hands and make sure the spices cover the entire surface of the chicken. Marinate for at least two hours. It is better to marinate the night before.

2. Breading the chicken marinated in coconut flour, heat oil in a deep fryer or saucepan to 190 °. Fry chicken being careful not to put too much at once so that the chicken becomes crispy. Cook 8 minutes on each side until chicken pieces are golden.

3. Rune thigh cut in two to make sure the meat is not pink in the interior.

Fall salad with pumpkin, cranberry and walnuts

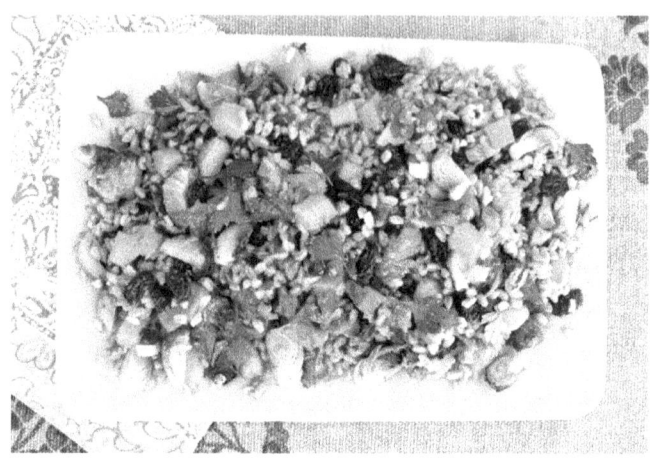

Ready in 15 minutes.

4 servings

Ingredients

- ✓ 3 cups butternut squash (butternut) or pumpkin
- ✓ 2 cups kale and / or chopped parsley
- ✓ ¼ of fresh lemon juice cup
- ✓ 1 tablespoon maple syrup table (or agave nectar)
- ✓ 1 tablespoon of hemp oil table (or other good oil)
- ✓ ¼ to ½ teaspoon of salt
- ✓ 2 tablespoons finely chopped onion table
- ✓ A small clove garlic, finely chopped
- ✓ 2 chopped fresh ginger root finely sliced
- ✓ About ½ cup chopped dried cranberries knife
- ✓ About ½ cup chopped walnuts knife

Preparation

1. Start by preparing the dressing in the bottom of a large salad bowl. Mix the lemon juice, oil, maple syrup, salt, onion, garlic and ginger.
2. To this dressing, add chopped greens so they imbibe well and they soften a little
3. Scatter nuts and dried cranberries, either directly in the bowl or individually on each serving.

Moroccan fava bean dip

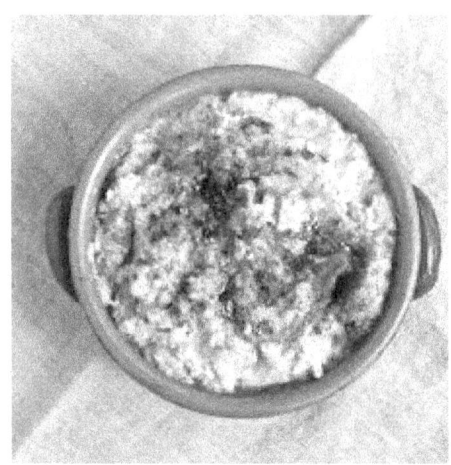

Prep time: 15 min

Cooking time: 40 min

6 servings

Ingredients

- 2 tbsps. vegetable oil
- 2 tbsps. cumin Powder
- 1 heaping teaspoon, harissa
- Salt to taste
- 2 teaspoons tahini
- 1 teaspoon paprika
- 3 cups water
- 1 tablespoon olive oil
- 2 cups soaked Split Fava Beans
- 1 lemon, zested and squeezed

Preparation

1. Get the pressure cooker heated at low heat and cook the garlic cloves up to the point they become golden.

2. Add garlic cloves, drained fava and vegetable oil and approximately three cups of water. Get the pressure cooker locked and adjust the cooker to low heat that can support high pressure. At the high pressure, cook for fifteen minutes.

3. With the natural release method, let the pressure be released. Get the cooking liquid drained.

4. Add tahini, harissa, cumin, and lemon zest. Puree the items using an immersion blender. Add salt for seasoning.

5. It is best served at room temperature.

Ligurian bean stew

Prep time: 15 min

Cooking time: 35 min

6 servings

Ingredients

- 1 heaping cup of dry Cannellini Beans
- 1 Garlic Clove
- 2-3 coriander seeds
- Extra Virgin Olive Oil
- 1 Tbsp. Olive Oil
- Ricotta Salata
- ½ cup Perlated Barley
- Tea Infuser
- 1 heaping cup of Chickpeas
- 4 cups or 1 L Water
- Salt and Pepper to Taste

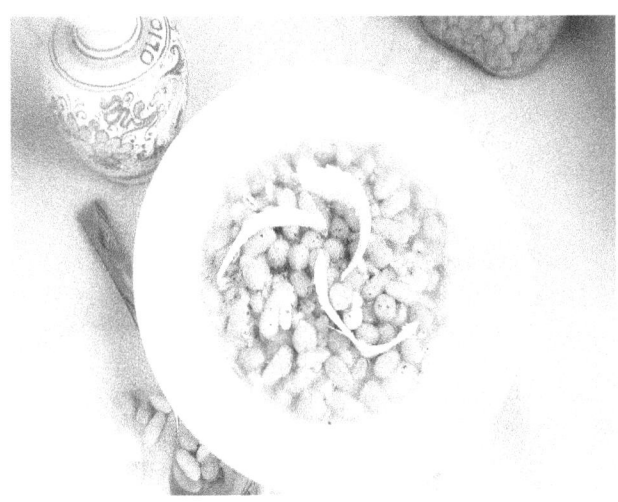

Preparation

1. Get each bean type soaked separately.

2. Get them rinsed then put them in a pressure cooker. Add garlic clove, water, salt, tea with spices, and barley.

3. Add one tablespoon of oil then add rinsed cannellini beans in the steamer basket.

4. Get the lid of the pressure cooker locked. Start by adjusting the heat to high and eventually to low once the highest pressure is reached. Under high pressure, allow it to cook for fifteen minutes.

5. Using the natural pressure release method, place the cooker in the burner, already cold and let the pressure come down on its own in the natural way.

6. Into the pot, add the beans from the steamer basket and get rid of the steamer basket.

7. Add pepper and salt and as you very well stir, allow it to rest for about five minutes. It is ready to serve and can be garnished before serving.

Spinach and artichoke DIP

Prep time: 10 min

Cooking time: 45 minutes

6 servings

Ingredients

- 2 crushed garlic cloves
- 2 cups artichke
- 1 onion (diced)
- 2 crushed garlic cloves
- 1 package frozen spinach already dried
- Artichoke oke hearts (chopped and drained)
- ¼ tablespoon black pepper (freshly ground)
- 1 tablespoon red wine vinegar
- 1/3 cup vegan mayonnaise

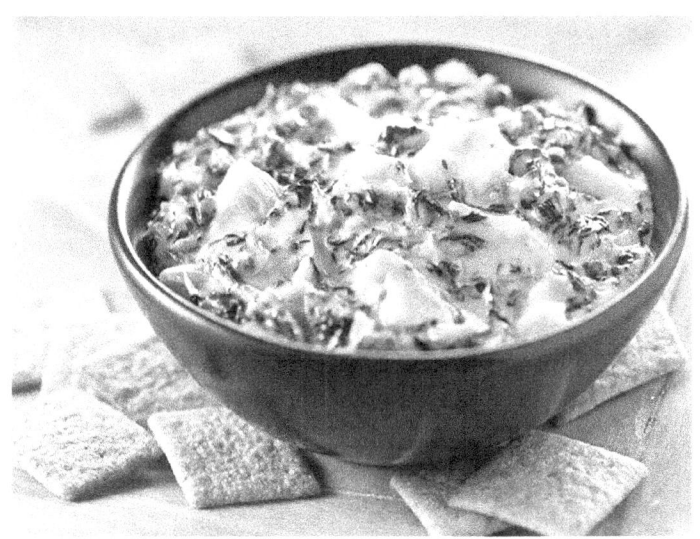

Preparation

1. Take thegarlic, onion, mayonnaise, vinegar,pepper,spinach, arichoke hearts, feta and and place all of them into the pressure cooker.

2. Stir until they are combined.

3. Cover it to cook under low heat and high pressure for approximately 25 minutes.

4. Remove the cover and stir again.

5. Cover once more and cook for about 10 minutes and allow for natural pressure release method.

Black beans in the pressure cooker

Prep time: 10 miNS

Cooking time: 40 min

4 servings

Ingredients

- 1 bay leaf

- 1 pound ham hock

- 2 minced cloves garlic

- 2 cups picked, rinsed, and dried black beans

- 1 medium onion, diced

- 6 cups of water

- 4 tbsps. extra-virgin olive oil

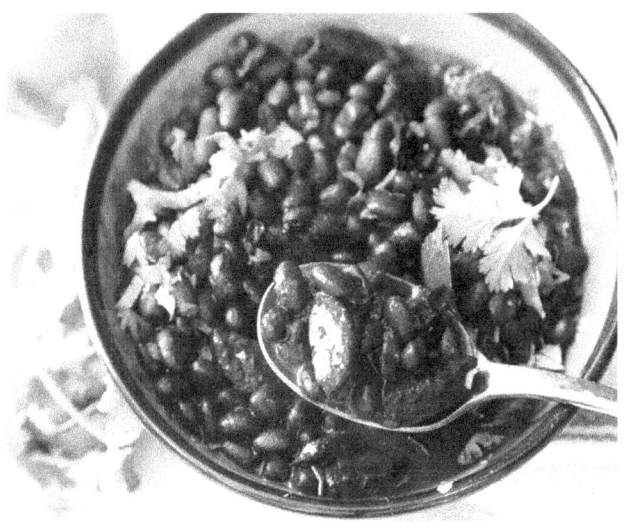

Preparation

1. Over low heat and high pressure, add 3 tablespoons of oil. Add onions and ham hock and get the onions cooked until they wilt and are brown. This could take about five minutes.

2. Add bay leaf and garlic and for one more minute, let them cook.

3. As you stir, add in beans. Add the oil that remained as well as water. Add again grinding pepper and a tablespoon of salt.

4. Adjust the cooker to high pressure and cover the cooker with the lid. Adjust the heat too to ensure a high pressure is maintained. Cook for twenty five minutes. Stop heating and allow for five minutes resting.

5. In accordance with the given instructions, let the steam be released. The beans by this time are tender. Get rid of the bay leaf. Add to the beans meat picked from the ham hock, get rid of the bone. Add seasoning as much as desired.

Mince and spinach salad

Ready in 10 minutes

4 servings

INGREDIENTS

- 150 g fresh spinach trimmed
- 150 g mince
- 1/2 cup unsalted nuts cashew
- 1 spring onion
- 2 cups raspberries
- 1/4 cup raspberry vinegar
- 2 c. tablespoons sugar choice
- 1/2 cup canola oil
- Salt and pepper

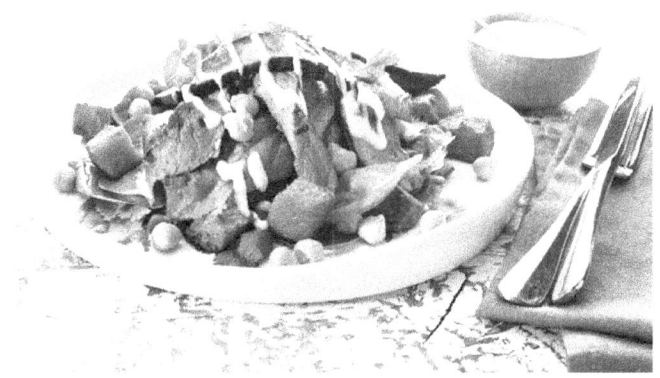

PREPARATION

1. In a bowl, mix the mince, spinach and apples.
2. For the dressing, in a pan, sweat the onion on low heat. Add the raspberries and mash.
3. Add vinegar and sugar, then reduce for 2 minutes. Book.
4. Once the preparation of vinaigrette has cooled, add the oil and whisk vigorously until smooth.
5. Place the dressing over the salad and garnish with cashews

Carpaccio avocado wild blueberry

Ready in 10 minutes.

4 servings

INGREDIENTS

- 4 young avocados
- 1 lime (juice)
- 1 pinch salt
- 250 g (250 ml or 1 1/2 cup) cottage cheese (optional)
- 250 ml fresh or frozen wild blueberries
- 5 ml (1 tsp.) Honey
- 1 pinch red pepper
- 375 ml alfalfa sprouts

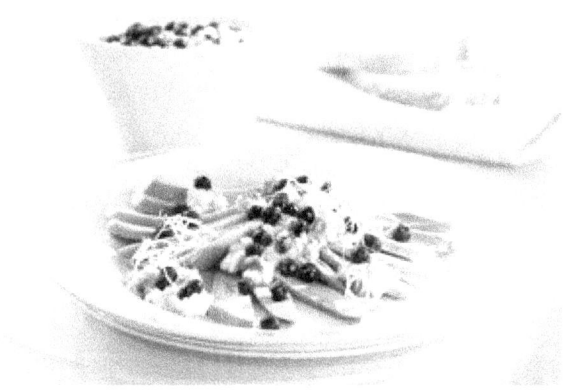

PREPARATION

1. Cut the avocados in half, peel and remove pits. Thinly slice and place on a plate. Drizzle with lime juice and salt.
2. Mix cottage cheese with wild blueberries (without the juice) and honey. Add red pepper to taste. Place the avocado slices and garnish with alfalfa sprouts.

DINNER RECIPES

Avocado stuffed with citrus salsa

Ready in 10 minutes.

2 portions

Ingredients

- 1 avocado
- 1 orange, peeled raw and cut into small cubes
- 1 pink grapefruit supreme, the supreme cut into small cubes
- About 2 tablespoons (30 mL) red onion, finely diced
- 1-2 tablespoons (15-30 ml) chopped fresh cilantro
- A pinch of pepper (or other good chili to taste)

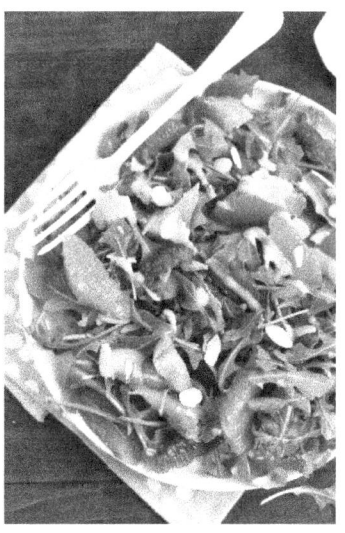

Preparation

1. Cut avocado lengthwise and remove the core.
2. Mix the citrus and seasonings and pour salsa in the avocados.
3. Serve on a bed of greens.

Spinach and apple sauce miso bench

Ready in 10 minutes.

2 servings

Ingredients

- 1 apple, peeled and cubed
- 2 large handfuls of spinach
- 1 tablespoon (15 mL) white miso
- 1 teaspoon (5 mL) tahini
- 1 teaspoon (5 mL) lemon juice
- 15 ml of water
- Freshly ground black pepper

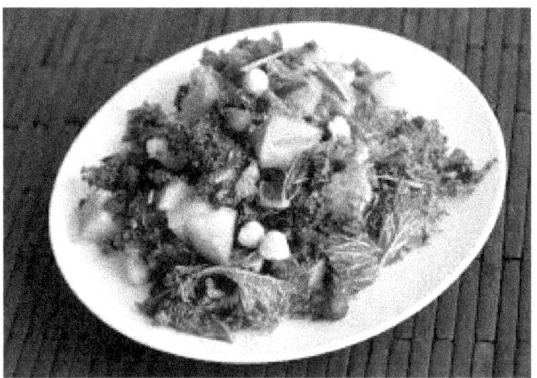

Preparation

1. Combine miso, tahini and lemon juice.
2. Add water little by little until a creamy sauce is attained.
3. Pour over spinach and apples, stir and serve immediately
4. Sprinkled with freshly ground pepper.

Ready in 4h.

4 servings.

Ingredients

- 2 pounds skinless, boneless chicken thighs
- 4 medium carrots, roughly shredded
- 4 tablespoons dry sherry
- 2 tablespoon soy sauce
- 2 tablespoon rice vinegar
- 2 teaspoon grated fresh ginger
- 1/2 teaspoon black pepper (ground)
- 5-15 - ounce can chicken broth
- 2 cups of water
- 18 - Ounce package frozen pea pods

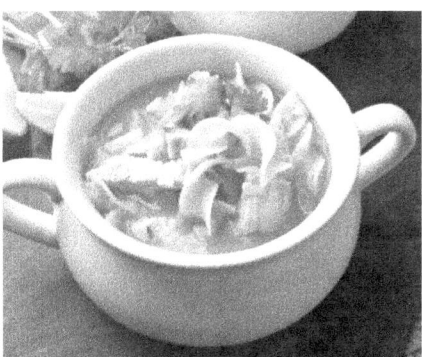

Directions

1. Combine chicken, carrots, sherry, the vinegar, ginger, and pepper on a slow cooker.
2. Stir in chicken broth and the water.
3. Cover and cook on high-heat setting for 3 to 4 hours.
4. Stir in noodles and pea pods.
5. Cover and cook for 10 to 15 minutes more or until noodles are tender.

Roast beef

Ready in 2 h. 20mins.

4 servings.

Ingredients

- 1 roast beef
- 4 tablespoons olive oil
- 1 tablespoon of herbs
- 1 pinch of salt

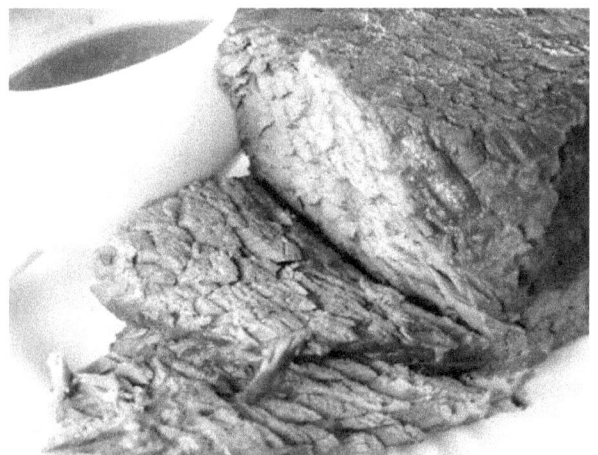

Preparation

1. Before you start cooking: mix the oil with herbs and salt. Brush in roasted over the entire surface. Roast in a skillet 2 minutes on all sides. Deglaze the pan with 100ml of water. Let stand.

2. Place the roast in a slow cooker. Insert the probe in the middle of the roast and cook at least 2 hours.

3. Enjoy!

Beef fillet

Ready in 5h. 15 mins.

 4 servings.

Ingredients

- ✓ 800 g beef tenderloin
  1 shallot
  2 tablespoons balsamic vinegar
  20 cl strong red wine
  50 cl beef funds
  100g butter

Preparation

1. Roast the fillet to the pan in very hot butter for about 5 minutes. Deglaze the butter with shallots finely chopped in a crockpot, add the red wine and reduce by half, then add balsamic vinegar and the veal stock.

2. Reduce again by half, then add 100g of butter you let melt and mix with the sauce.
   Pour the beef fillet with the sauce and let it cook for 3 hours for perfect cooking.

3. Enjoy

Fried pork with noodles

Ready in 1h.

4 servings.

Ingredients

- ✓ 150 g Chinese noodles
  200g pork loin
  90 g of soy
  2 tablespoons soy sauce
  1 tablespoon honey
  2 handfuls of black mushrooms
  4 tablespoons olive oil

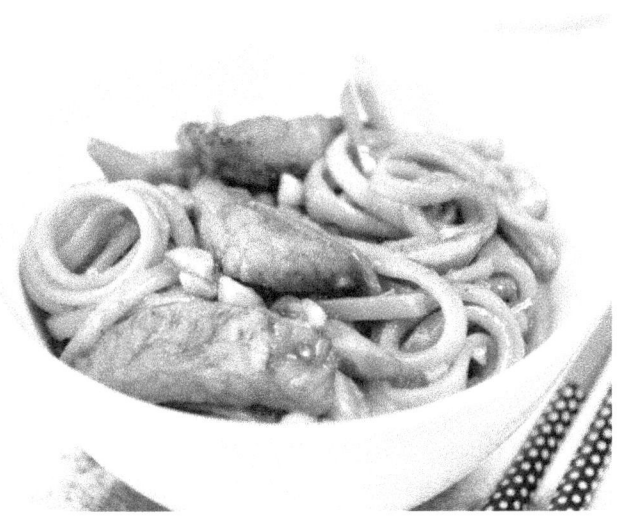

Preparation

1. Cut the meat and the mushrooms.
   In a slow cooker, put the oil and meat leave covered as long as the meat cooks, stir regularly.
   Cook pasta in a saucepan. Add the soy sauce, honey, mushrooms.

2. Allow 5 minutes and when the pasta is ready, add them to the slow cooker. Cook for 10 mins.

Gratin salmon and spinach

Prep time 5mins.

Cooking time 40min.

6 servings.

Ingredients

- 150 grams of smoked salmon

- A large bowl of cooked spinach (revenues in butter)

- 100 grams of cheese cream cheese with garlic and herbs

- A handful of grated cheese

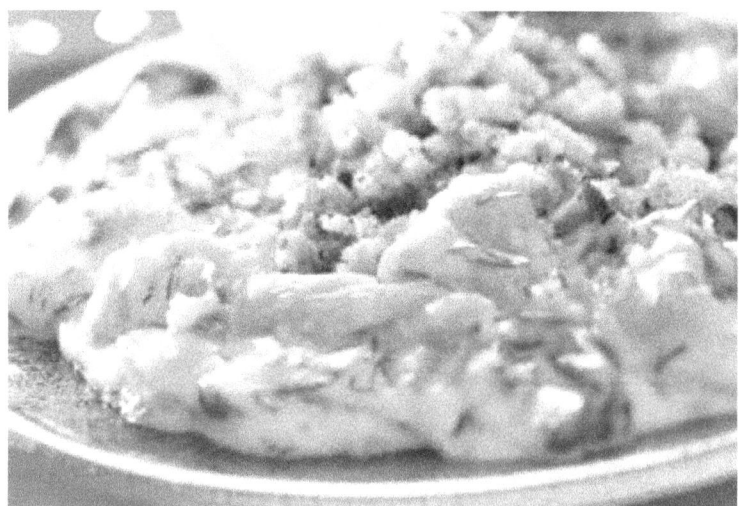

Preparation

- ✓ Mix the spinach with cream cheese, gently add the smoked salmon. Put in a baking dish and sprinkle with grated cheese.

- ✓ Put in a hot oven.

Meatzza

Prep time 3mins.

Cooking time 25min.

1 portion.

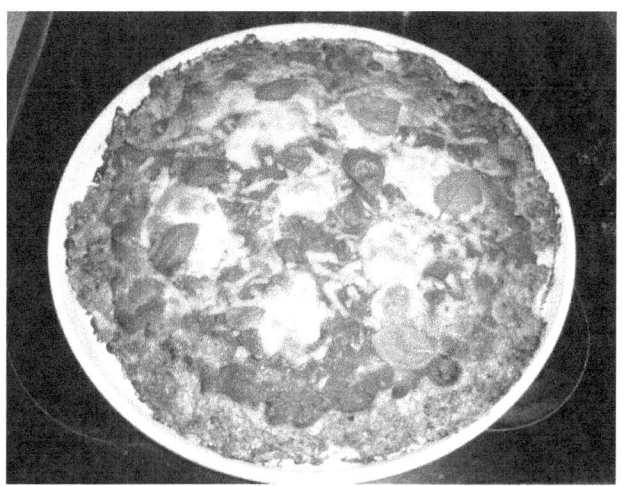

Ingredients

- 2 eggs

- A small bowl of tomato sauce

- 500 grams of minced meat

- Half a pepper cut into washer

- Half onion cut into thin slices

- 2 tablespoons grated Parmesan cheese

- 150 grams of grated cheese

- Salt and pepper

- Tabasco

Preparation

1. Salt and pepper the chopped meat, add two beaten eggs, 2 tablespoons grated Parmesan and shape as a pizza dough in a baking dish.

2. Garnish with tomato sauce, peppers, onions, a few drops of Tabasco sauce and grated cheese.

3. Bake for 20 minutes at 200 degrees. Serve with a salad.

Bone broth

Prep time 3mins.

Cooking time 35min.

5 servings.

Ingredients:

- 1 kg of ' bone beef or a chicken carcass
- A sprig of thyme
- 2 bay leaves
- A beautiful celery
- A small bunch of parsley
- 5 peppercorns (or pepper)
- 2 cloves of garlic
- 1 carrot cut into thick trogons
- Half of a medium onion
- 1 leek cut into thick sections
- A teaspoon salt
- 4 tbsps. cider vinegar
- 2 tablespoons chopped parsley

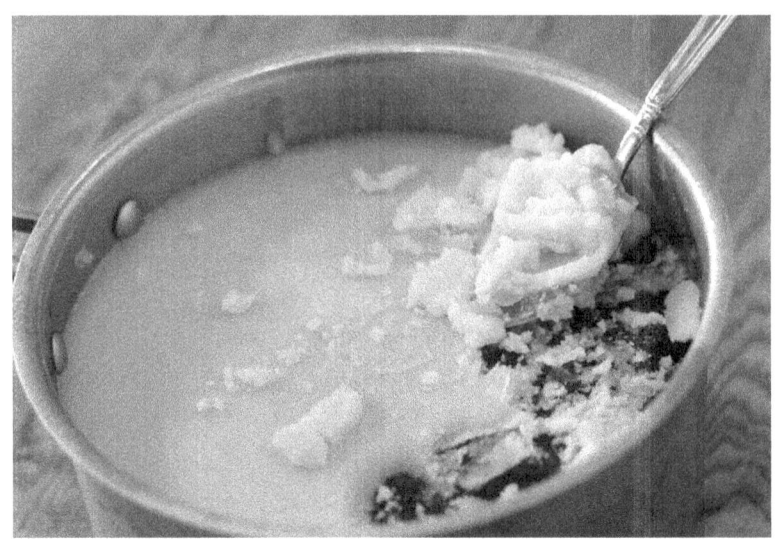

Preparation

- ✓ In a Dutch oven or casserole, put the oil to heat; add the bones, pods of garlic, peppercorns, salt and vegetables. Make a bouquet garni with thyme, bay leaf, parsley and celery, put in the pan, cover with water and cook over low heat for half past one.

- ✓ Pass the bones and vegetables in a colander to keep only the liquid.

- ✓ Sprinkle with chopped parsley before serving.

Marrakesh vegetable curry

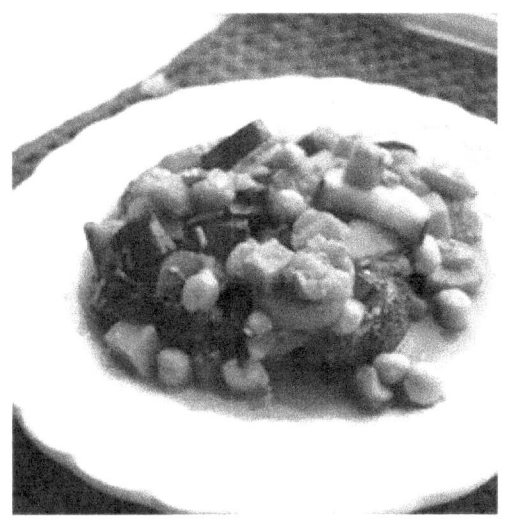

Prep time: 15 min |

Cooking time: 40 min

6 servings

Ingredients

- 1 teaspoon ground cinnamon

- 2 carrots, chopped

- 1 cup orange juice

- 1 can of drained garbanzo beans

- 1 zucchini, sliced

- 1 red bell pepper, chopped

- 4 minced garlic cloves

- 1 tbsp of curry powder

- 1 onion, chopped

- 1/2 tablespoon sea salt

- 1 green bell pepper, chopped

- 3/4 teaspoon cayenne pepper

- 1 medium cubed eggplant

- 1 teaspoon grated ginger

- 2 tablespoons raisins

- 1/4 cup blanched almond

- 2 teaspoons ground turmeric

- 1 sweet potato, peeled and cubed

- 10 ounces spinach

- 6 tablespoons olive oil

Preparation

1. Heat oil in a pressure cooker. Add sweet potatoes and carrots then cook for a few minutes.

2. Add raisins, orange juice and chickpeas then cook for twelve minutes.

3. Add zucchini, onion, eggplant, bell peppers and garlic then cook for extra ten minutes.

4. Add curry powder, sea salt, ginger, spinach, turmeric, cinnamon, and cayenne. Cook for six minutes.

5. It is best served with overcooked white rice

Vegan Garlic cauliflower and mashed potatoes

Prep time: 10 min

Cooking time: 45mins

6 serving

Ingredients

- 3 cups water

- 1 teaspoon salt

- 1 tablespoon vegan butter

- 1 bay leaf

- 4 large garlic cloves, peeled

- Salt and Pepper

- 1 head of cauliflower

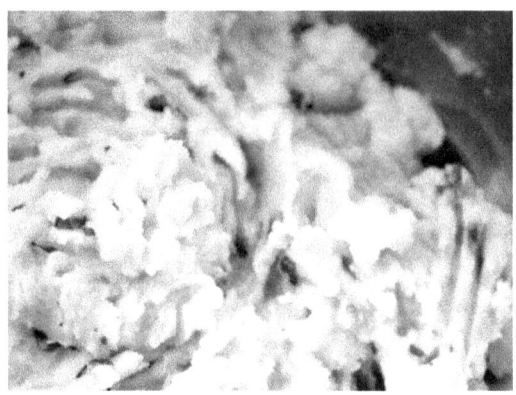

Preparation

1. Make florets out of the cauliflower then put them into the pressure cooker. Add bay leaf, garlic cloves, salt and water. While covered, cook for about 35 minutes on high pressure and low heat. Get out the bay leaf and garlic cloves.

2. Get rid of the water. Take your butter and add it then allow it to melt as you allow for natural pressure release method.

3. Mash the cauliflower using a potato masher. Season with pepper and salt. Use green onions or chives to serve.

Moroccan Chickpea soup

Prep time: 15 min

Cooking time:

6 servings

Ingredients

- 1 /2 teaspoon ground ginger
- 1/2 teaspoon ground coriander
- 1 chopped onion
- ½ cup chopped salt celery (with leaves)
- 1 15 ounce can diced and fire roasted tomatoes
- 1/2-teaspoon cinnamon
- 1/4 teaspoon ground cumin
- 3 cups of vegetable broth
- 1/4 teaspoon cayenne pepper
- 2 peeled medium carrots peeled (chopped)
- 1 diced and peeled medium sweet potato
- 2 cups seeded bell peppers (chopped)
- 1 9-ounce bag baby spinach
- 2 15-ounce cans drained chickpeas
- 1/2 teaspoon ground ginger

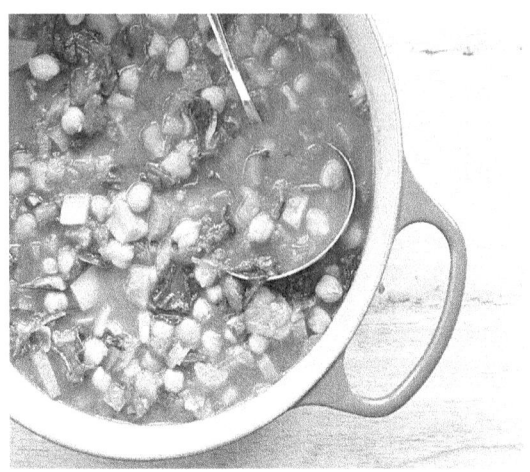

Preparation

1. Add tomatoes, spices, Vegetable broth, celery, bell peppers, carrots and chickpeas to the pressure cooker. The pressure cooker should be adjusted to high pressure for 30 minutes.

2. After approximately 20 minutes, add sweet potato.

3. Adjust the pressure cooker to relatively low heat and add spinach as you stir cooking them for three minutes until they wilt. The food is ready. Use quick pressure release method.

Vegan split pea and sweet potato soup

Ready after 1 hour 35 minutes,

2 servings

Ingredients

- 4 cups vegetable broth

- Cayenne pepper

- 7 whole green cardamom pods

- 1 medium yellow onion, chopped

- 1/2 teaspoon ground cumin

- 1 teaspoon garam masala

- Lemon juice

- 1 tablespoon ghee (clarified butter) or canola oil

- 1/8 teaspoon fine sea salt

- 1 medium sweet potato, peeled and cut into 1/2-inch slices

- Ground black pepper, to taste

- 1 cup yellow split peas

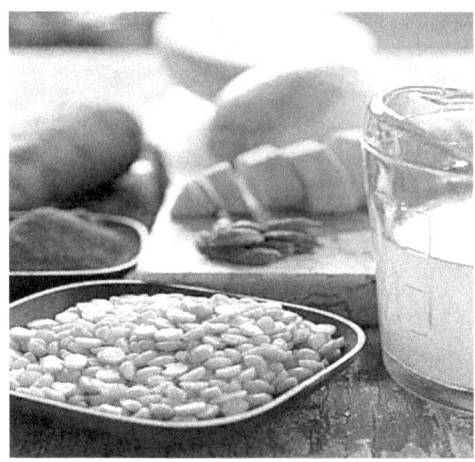

Preparation

1. Soak peas overnight and drain as you rinse them.

2. Boil the vegetable broth in a pot using a stove. Add sweet potatoes slices, soaked beans and cardamom pods. Adjust the heat such that there is just a simmer and ensure you cover for approximately one hour.

3. Take your skillet and in it heat the ghee.

4. Add garam masala, onions and cumin and for about ten minutes, cook as you stir. Once the peas and sweet potatoes are tender, take your spiced onions and add them to the pot. Cook for five minutes as you stir.

5. Get out cardamom pods and using cayenne, lemon, and salt, season the soup to taste.

Indian Spiced chard with tofu

Ready after 40 minutes

4 servings

Ingredients

- 1teaspoon cumin powder

- 1 chopped onion

- 3 cloves of garlic

- 1 tomato (chopped)

- 1 teaspoon garam masala

- 0.24 liters of water

- 20 grams tarnishing cilantro (chopped)

- 3 tablespoons of olive oil

- 17 leaves rainbow chard

- 1 tablespoon minced ginger

- 1 teaspoon turmeric

- ½ teaspoon red chili flakes

- 1 teaspoon kosher salt

- 1 block cubed extra firm tofu

- 0.035 kilograms of garnishing roasted cashews

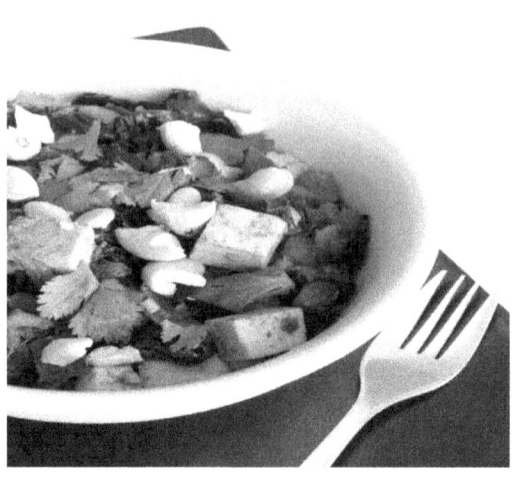

Preparation

1. Take your chard of stalks, rip them of the leaves and keep them aside. Take again the chard leaves and chop them into pieces of bite size. Before chopping the stalks, wash them very well and rinse them.

2. Heat the olive oil in a pressure cooker. Add garlic, onions, and ginger and cook them for three minutes until they turn golden brown. Add the already cleaned up chard stalks and cook for two minutes.

3. Add garam masala, red chili flakes, salt, and turmeric and then cook until fragrant.

4. Take your tomatoes and add them cooking them until fully crushed.

5. On medium heat, add and cook the chard leaves and for about 2 minutes, cook them until wilting of the leaves is observed.

6. Reduce pressure a little bit after adding water and tofu and allowing them to boil.

7. Cook on that low heat for 20 minutes until the flavors are melded and chard cooks down. Allow pressure to be released naturally.

Black eyed pea soup

Preparation time: 10 minutes

Cooking time: 10 minutes

5 servings

Ingredients

- 1 cup of black eyed peas, soaked overnight

- 2 cups of yellow split peas, soaked with the peas

- 1 cup millet

- 1 half onion, put to equal about 1 cup

- 2 stalks celery, diced

- 2 carrots, diced

- 2 bay leaves

- 2 sprigs of thyme and a small sprig of rosemary or 2 teaspoons dried thyme.

- All purpose , no salt, herb and spice seasoning or seasoning of your choice 1 to 2 tablespoons

- 6 cups homemade vegetable stock

- 4 cups or more chopped greens

- 1 ½ cups tomato sauce or diced or crushed tomatoes

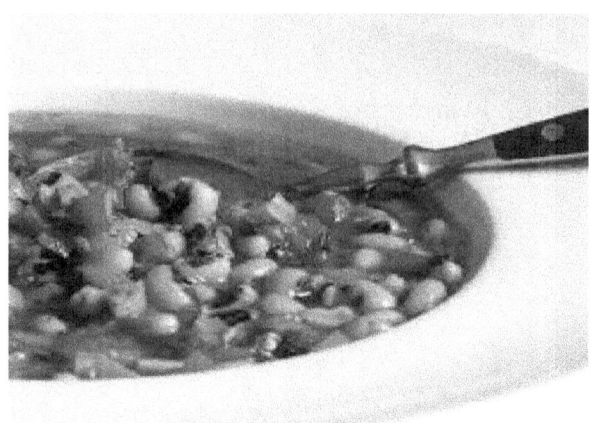

Preparation

1. Dry the onion, carrot and celery for a few minutes.

2. Put the drained black eyed and split peas and the millet in one container.

3. Mix them with the bay leaves, thyme, rosemary seasoning and the stock.

4. Cover the pressure cooker with the pressure cooker lid on the pressure cooker and bring to high pressure for 10 minutes.

5. After the 10 minutes are over, let the pressure come down by itself. Add the chopped greens and stir well. Greens can cook with absolutely low heat so they cook with the heat from the soup to cook from. When not available, let the soup boil for one more minute and without stirring. Add the diced tomatoes and serve.

Apple crumble

Prep time 20mins.

Cooking time 25min.

6 servings.

Ingredients

- 1 kg of Canada gray apples

- 1/2 lemon

- 125 g of buckwheat flour

- 125g ground almonds

- 100g margarine with Omega-3

- 100 g sugar

- 1 c. c. ground cinnamon

- Olive oil

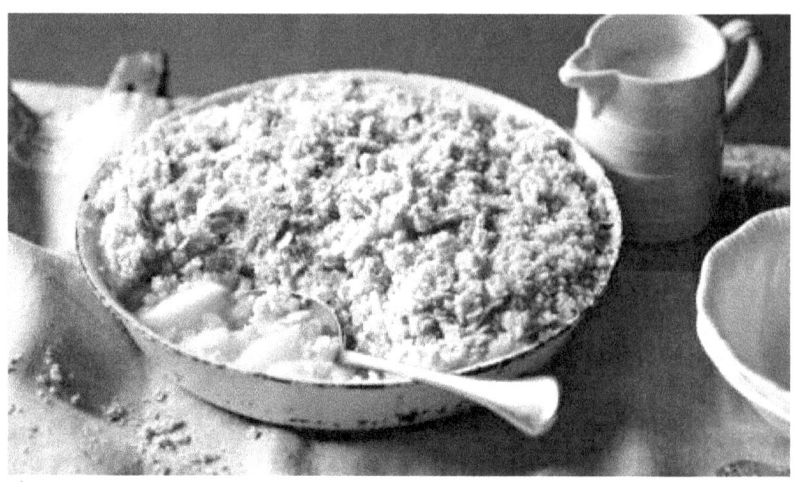

Preparation

1. Preheat oven to 180-200 ° C (th. 6 -7). Oil a baking dish (preferably Pyrex). Peel and cut apples into thin slices. Put them in the dish and sprinkle with lemon juice.

2. Bake for 10 to 15 minutes (possibly stir halfway through cooking). Meanwhile, put buckwheat flour, ground almonds, sugar and margarine in a bowl. Add cinnamon.

3. Mix for coarse sand. Remove the dish from the oven, mix some apples and crumble over the pastry. Bake 10 minutes, then turn off and let the dish in the oven for another 10 minutes. Serve warm.

Red cabbage cooked with apples and chestnuts

Prep time 20mins.

Cooking time 20min.

4 servings.

Ingredients

- 1 red cabbage

- 2 apple tart flesh

- 200 g of natural chestnut

- 1 onion

- 1 c. to s. olive oil

- Thyme

- 5 bay leaves

- Herb salt

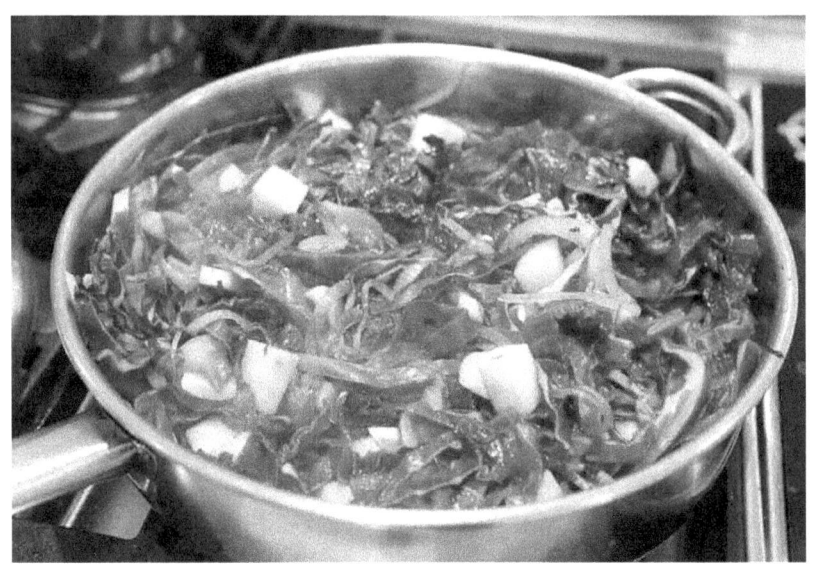

Preparation

1. Remove the hard core cabbage then cut it into thin strips.

2. Add the bay leaves, cover the cabbage strips sprinkled with thyme and some salt with herbs. Bake about 10 minutes.

3. Meanwhile, in a saucepan, melt over very low heat, without browning, onion finely chopped in olive oil and remaining thyme.

4. Add the cabbage and chestnuts, mix then put over the apples cut into thick slices. When the potatoes are cooked, serve immediately.

Vegetable grated cheese

Prep time 8mins.

Cooking time 22min.

4 servings.

Ingredients

- 500 ml of water
- 40 g of chopped tomatoes
- 35 g of raw almonds or cashews (or sunflower seeds)
- 1/4 c. c. garlic powder
- 1/2 c. c. onion powder
- 1/2 c. to s. salt
- 1/2 c. to s. lemon juice
- 2 c. to s. arrowroot
- 25g flaked yeast

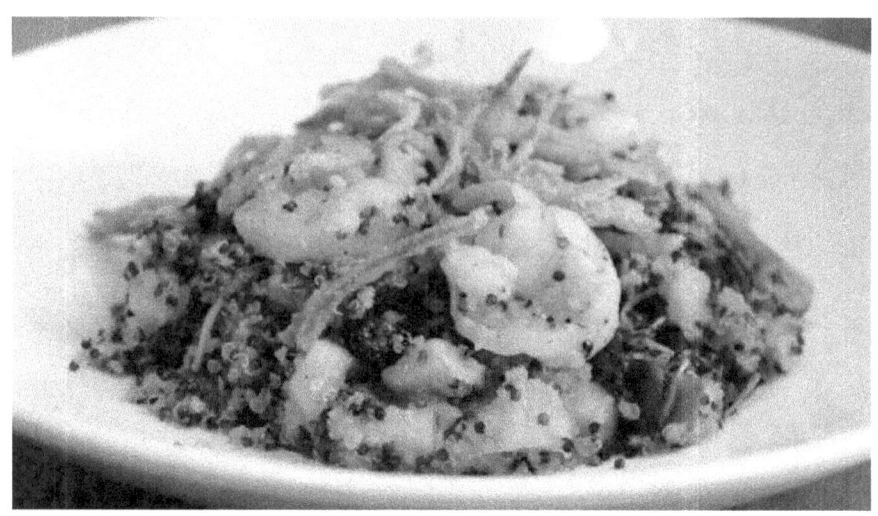

Preparation

1. Mix all ingredients in a blender until the mixture obtained is smooth.

2. Then put the mixture in a saucepan and cook over low heat stirring constantly until it thickens.

Squash crumble, fennel and onions with garlic

Prep time 20mins.

Cooking time 40min.

4 servings.

Ingredients

- 500g butternut squash
- 2 fennel bulbs
- 2 onions
- ½ glass 25cl vegetable broth
- Thyme, herb salt
- 2 pinches of grated nutmeg
- 2 large garlic cloves
- 125 g of rice flour
- 50 g of finely ground nuts
- Olive oil

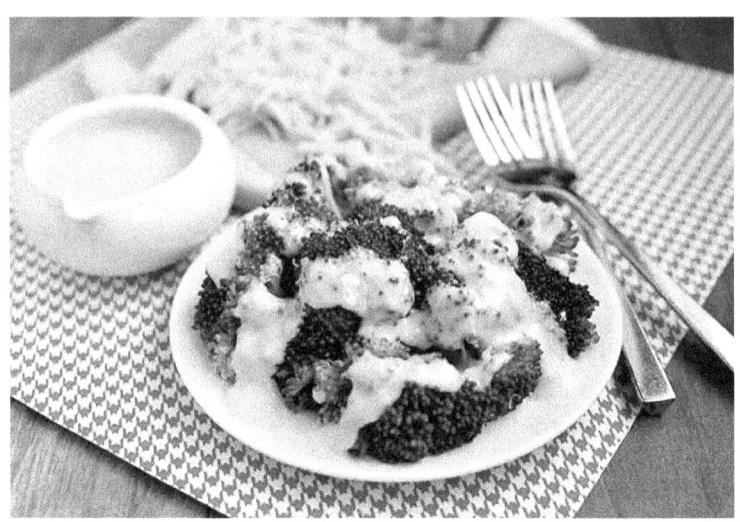

Preparation

1. Peel and cut squash into large "fries" very thick, thinly slice the fennel and onions.

2. Pour the vegetable stock into the bottom of a glass baking dish and garnish the dish by inserting rows of squash, onion and fennel.

3. Tighten rows. Drizzle lightly with olive oil. Prepare the crumble topping by mixing in a bowl the flour and nuts which added little by little olive oil until you notice the consistency of lumpy dough that kneads your fingertips.

4. Spread nutmeg, chopped garlic cloves and crumble over the vegetables. Bake at 110 ° C and cook until vegetables are melting.

Venison with mushrooms and nuts

Prep time 25mins.

Cooking time 45min.

2 servings.

Ingredients

- 250g fillet of venison

- 100g mushrooms

- 25 g walnuts / pine nuts

- Chopped parsley

- ½ onion

- 1 garlic clove

- 300 g shallots

- 200 ml port

- Cinnamon

- 300 ml red wine

- 100 g of honey

- Olive oil

- Salt

- pepper

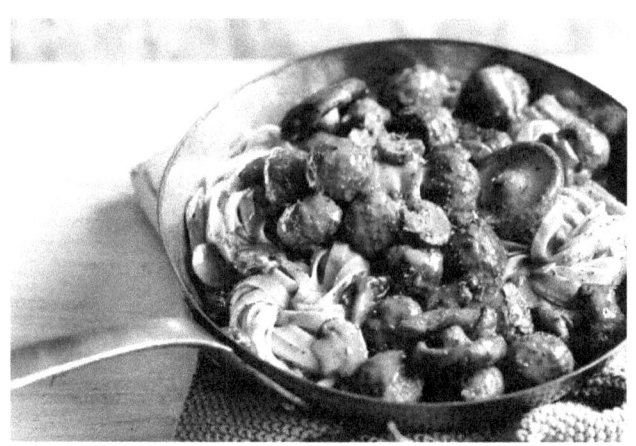

Preparation

1. Make confit slowly over low heat the shallots and garlic in wine mixture, port, honey, cinnamon and seasoning for 1 hour.

2. Place the piece of meat in the marinade once the cooled mixture. Fry the mushrooms in olive oil with chopped onion, walnuts and pine nuts and season. Roast meat piece at 200 ° C for 8 minutes.

3. Heat garlic and shallots and use the juice of wine to water the piece of meat after cooking and make a sauce.

4. Serve the dish by arranging around the piece of meat the mixture of mushrooms, shallots, garlic, parsley, and drizzle with sauce just before serving.

DESSERTS

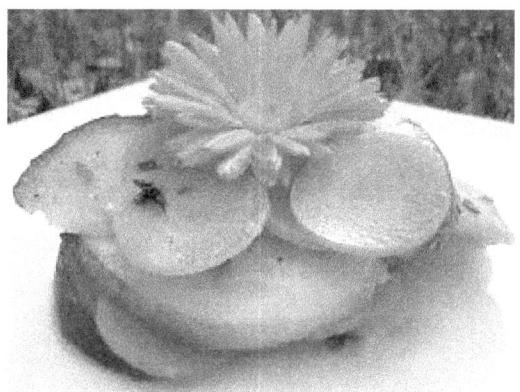

Carrots and peaches with fresh thyme

Ready in 35 minutes. 2 servings

Ingredients

- ✓ 1 unpeeled peach into thin slices
- ✓ 1 unpeeled carrot cut into very thin slices
- ✓ 2 tablespoons (30 mL) fresh orange juice
- ✓ leaves fresh thyme
- ✓ 1 pinch of salt
- ✓ 1 shot of pepper mill

Preparation

1. Mix all ingredients gently. It is important that the carrot is sliced thin enough to be crispy without being tough.
2. Let stand at least 30 minutes before serving.

Raffaello

Ready in 10 minutes.

5 servings

Ingredients:

- 1 cup raw cashew nuts
- 1/2 cup grated coconut
- 1/2 lemon juice
- 3 cases of water
- 1 pinch of vanilla seeds
- 3 dates
- 15 almonds

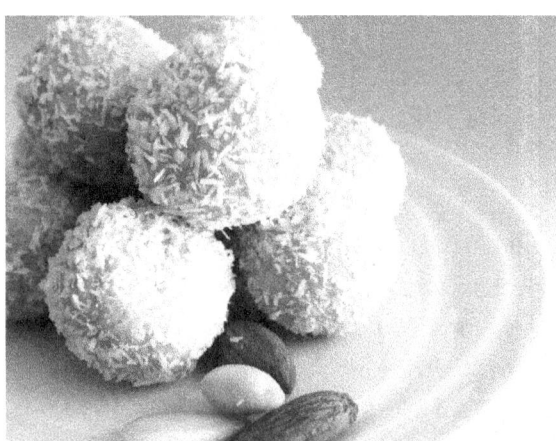

Preparation:

1. Soak cashews for a few hours and be sure to choose raw nuts, not those roasted and salted.
2. After that drain time and put all the ingredients except almonds in a blender to grind all the finely as possible.
3. Form small balls with your hands, with these quantities make fifteen balls; insert into each ball an almond. Looking to give a nice round shape and then roll in shredded coconut.

Brick raw carrot

Ready in 5 hours. 3 servings

Ingredients for the base:

- 200 gr almonds
- 5-600 grams of carrots
- 150g of dried apricots
- 70 ml water
- grated zest of one lemon
- 60 gr grated coconut
- 1 tsp. vanilla
- 1 cinnamon case
- 1/4 tsp. of powdered cloves
- 1/4 teaspoon ginger powder
- 1/4 tsp. salt
- 50g walnuts
- 70g raisins

Ingredients for the cream:

- Cases of coconut grated zest and sugar with a half a lemon
- 60g cashew nut
- 3 apricots
- 1 teaspoon vanilla
- 30 ml water

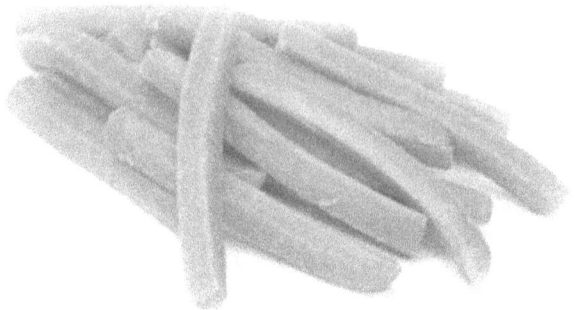

Preparation:

1. To the base, cut dried apricots into small pieces dried apricots and soak in 70 ml of water for 3 hours to obtain a smooth cream.
2. Grind the almonds and cut carrots and mash until smooth. Mix whole almonds, carrots, apricot cream, lemon zest, coconut, salt and spices
3. Chop nuts with a knife, combine nuts and grapes and mix thoroughly.
4. Share the unit into two halves and pour each portion into a loaf pan lined with parchment paper. Keep molds in the freezer.
5. For the cream: just mix the ingredients together. Spread each a layer of cream over the molds, booking again in the freezer for two hours. After this time combine both preparations in a single mold, squeeze a little and leave in the fridge overnight.

Truffles flood

Ready in 25 minutes.

25-28 truffles

Ingredients

- 1 cup walnut (135 g)
- 1/4 cup plus 1/2 cup of oatmeal (70 g)
- 1/6 cup coconut oil
- 1/6 cup agave syrup or rice malt
- Cane sugar
- Cinnamon powder

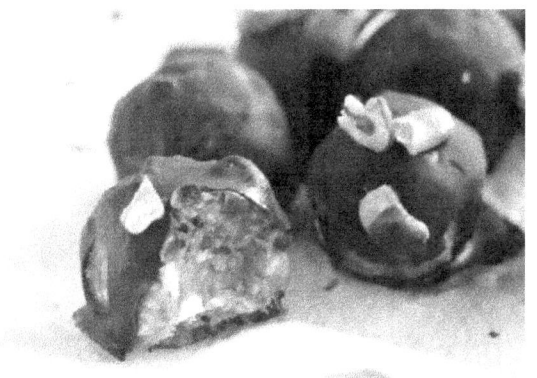

Preparation:

1. Grind 25 grams of oatmeal (1/4 cup) in the blender
2. Add Brazil nuts and grind again to push out oil
3. Compress the nuts slightly to the unit.
4. Transferred the mixture into a bowl, add the other 45 g flakes (1/4 cup), agave syrup and softened coconut oil.
5. Mix well and form pellets and a mixture of sugar and cinnamon and set aside in the

Fridge

Mushroom Salad

Ready in 15 minutes.6 servings

Ingredients

- 500 gr of Paris mushrooms
- Edible flowers like daisies
- Some flat parsley leaves
- For salad dressing:
- 2 cm fresh ginger root
- 1/2 shallot
- 10 large parsley leaves
- 2 tablespoons of cider vinegar
- Salt
- 6 tablespoons of virgin olive oil

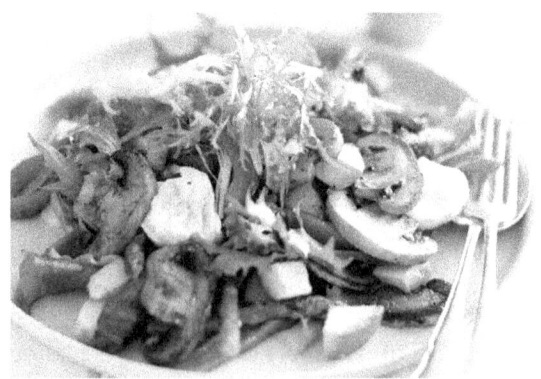

Preparation:

1. Cut up mushrooms, pass quickly under the tap to remove any soil, cut into thin slices and arrange in a dish, sprinkle with parsley and flowers.
2. Prepare the vinaigrette by mixing well all ingredients, marinate a bit and serve

Ready in 10 minutes.

4 servings.

Ingredients

- 250 g. carrots,
- Orange juice
- 15 g. water of orange flowers (1 cap)
- Salt, herbs (optional)

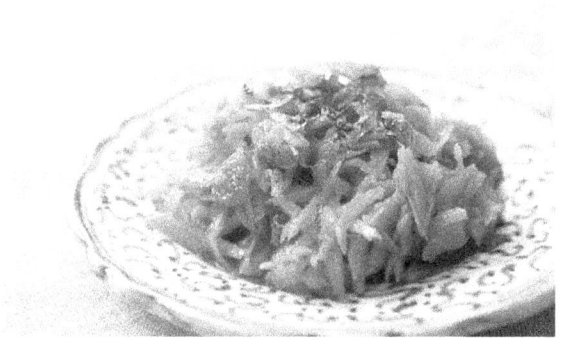

Preparation

1. Peel the carrots and grate them.
2. Squeeze the juice from the orange. Mix the ingredients.
3. Serve chilled.

Hummus.

Ready in 10 minutes

1 serving.

INGREDIENTS

- 1 cup of sesame butter
- 1/4 cup water
- Lemon juice
- 2 cloves garlic
- 1/2 c. Salt tea
- 1 cup mashed chickpeas

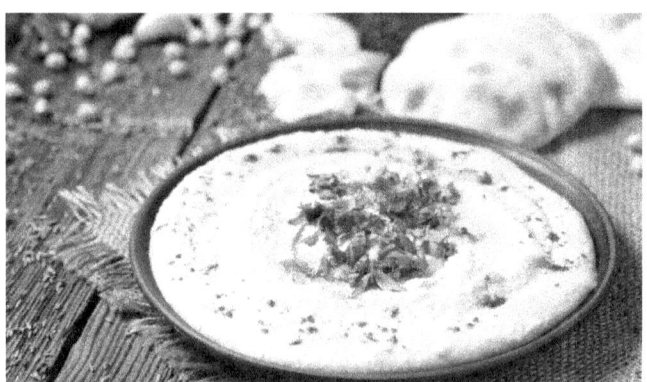

PREPARATION

1. Mix the oil in the sesame butter jar before measuring.
2. Add water and juice.
3. Crush the garlic with the salt and add to mixture.
4. Add chick peas mashed.

Flaxseed and honey.

Ready in 125 minutes.

4 portions

INGREDIENTS

- ✓ 1 cup flax seeds
- ✓ 1/4 cup honey

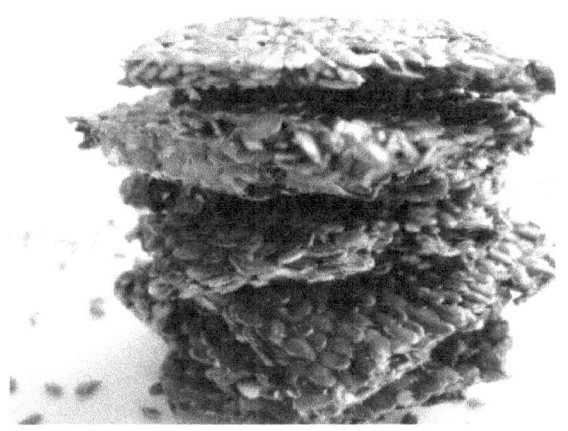

PREPARATION

1. Leave hydrate overnight flax seeds in 2 times their volume of water. The seeds will form mucilage, a kind of sticky liquid that can release their nutrients (enzymes, omega 3, and trace elements).
2. Add honey to the paste and spread the dough on parchment paper. Bake at the lowest temperature of the oven for 24 hours.
3. Cut dough to taste and serve

Super Honey bars

Ready in 20 mins.18 portions.

INGREDIENTS

- 125 ml unpasteurized honey
- 500 ml unsalted seeds (sunflower seeds, almonds, pumpkin seeds, currants)
- 125 ml unsalted peanuts
- 125 ml tamari almonds or kind
- 250 ml Sweetened Dried Cranberries
- 125 ml raisins

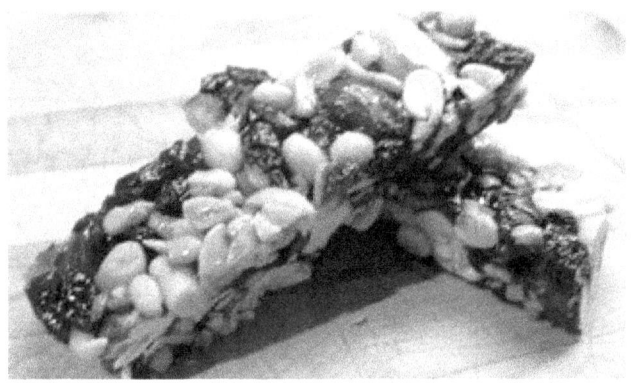

PREPARATION

1. Boil honey in a large pot for about 7 minutes. Remove from heat. Add cranberries and raisins and mix well. Add the rest and mix to coat all nuts, seeds and fruits.
2. Remove and spread the mixture into an oiled square. Press with a square of wax paper.
3. Compact few times to equalize well. Let stand about 15 minutes.
4. Remove the paper and place on a plate. Cut into 2, then 9 to 18 equal portions. Put each bar in a piece of transparent plastic and wrap. Keep cool.

Pink cream buckwheat.

Ready in 10 minutes.

2 Servings

Ingredients

- ✓ ½ cup whole buckwheat, not roasted and hulled
- ✓ 1 tablespoon of flaxseed
- ✓ ⅔ cupcashew milk
- ✓ ½ banana
- ✓ ¼ cup fresh or frozen raspberries
- ✓ 1 pitted date
- ✓ ¼ teaspoon ground vanilla
- ✓ 1 tablespoon of hemp seed
- ✓ 1 tablespoon of chia seeds
- ✓ 1 teaspoon of raw cocoa nibs
- ✓ Some fresh fruits
- ✓ Some nuts and seeds (almonds, cashews, Brazil nuts, pumpkin seeds)

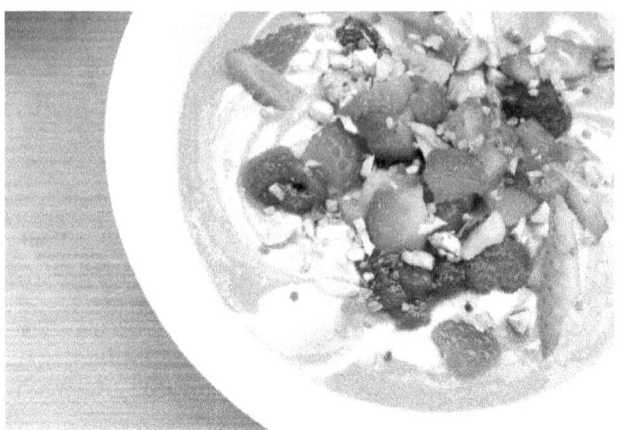

Preparation

1. The night before, soak the buckwheat seeds in a large bowl of cold water.
2. The next day, rinse thoroughly with clean water. This step serves to remove the mucilage, a viscous liquid produced by the hardened buckwheat.
3. In the bowl of a high speed blender, add all the ingredients of the cream and mix until smooth and creamy.
4. Pour into a bowl and place the gasket starting with hemp, chia, cocoa, and nuts and fresh fruit.

If you liked this book you may like these other books from Henry White

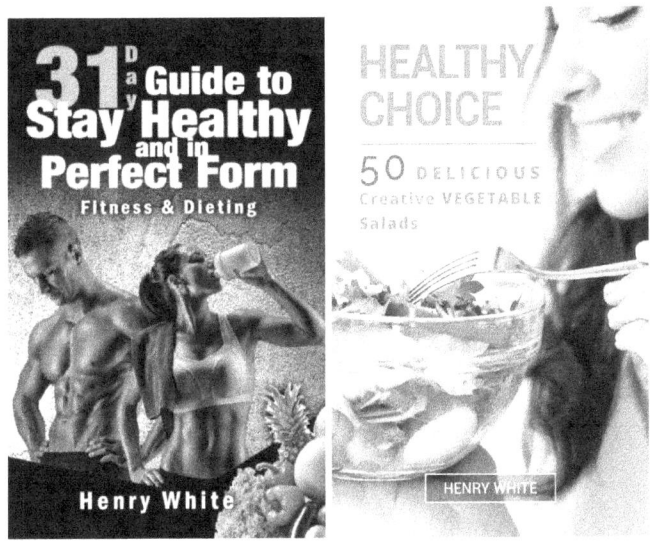

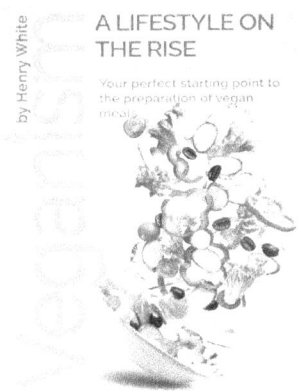

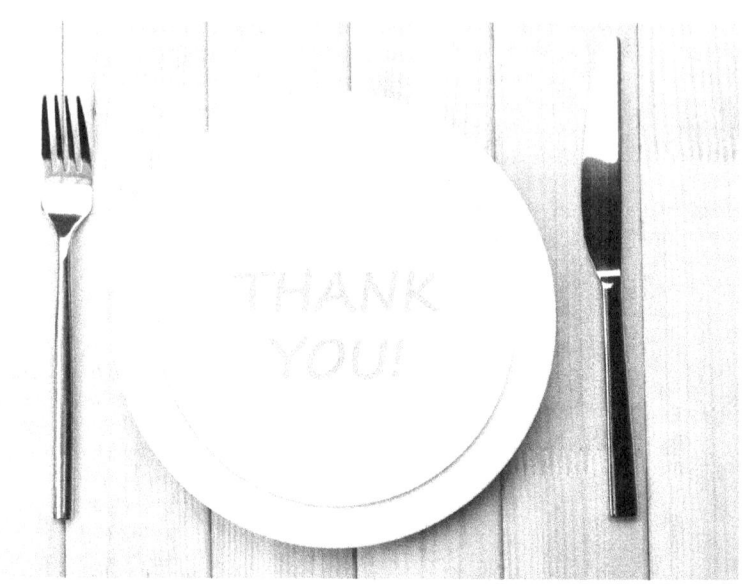

Did you enjoy this book?

I want to thank you for purchasing and reading this book. I really hope you got a lot out of it.

Can I ask a quick favor through?

If you enjoyed this book I would really appreciate ii if you could leave me an honest review on Amazon.

www.ingramcontent.com/pod-product-compliance
Lightning Source LLC
Chambersburg PA
CBHW072206280526
45788CB00002B/898